IRON ISOMETRICS

By Steve Justa

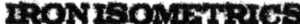

Iron Isometrics
© 2014, Steve Justa, William B Jeffries,
Strongerman Productions LLC, All Rights Reserved
ISBN 978-1-312-69683-9

Iron Isometrics

I dedicate this book to the Master Creator of the Universe and the supreme knowledge that's out there.

My goal with this training book is to provide to-the-point, in as few words as possible, a well-rounded, useful look at Isometric training.

Table of Contents

Steve's Story with Isometrics Today

Steve Justa spent nearly his entire adult life being single mindedly focused on gaining strength. He was obsessed with being as strong as and like some of the old time strongmen. In fact he did reach some completely legendary feats such as a 4,800 pound backlift, a 2,100 pound hand and thigh lift, shouldering a 330 pound barrel and many, many more feats of strength and endurance.

During his career, Steve would manipulate his bodyweight up and down depending on the goal he wanted. In his last push for some of the really heavy old time lifts, he pushed his bodyweight up to between 360-380 pounds and stayed there for nearly ten years. Even though he was incredibly strong and in good shape, carrying that bodyweight for that long was just too much. Steve began to feel badly and didn't know why. He suddenly got weak. One day he stepped off a curb and his leg buckled and he knew something was wrong. At that point he had some of the strongest legs on the planet, but even that wasn't enough to push him to go to a doctor, he's not that kind of a guy.

Steve's bodyweight began to rapidly drop and he went from being a 380 pound monster to 210 pounds in eight months. This nearly ended tragically. Even though he was drinking several gallons of water per day during that period (among other things), his stubbornness prevented him from seeing a doctor. During that time, his feet suffered the most and soon enough he wasn't able to walk or stand on his toes. Going from some of the strongest legs in the world to such a serious weakness in just eight months was finally enough for Steve to pay a visit to a doctor.

After many tests, Steve was diagnosed with Type 2 diabetes. His blood sugar level was 800 and the doctor told him he was lucky to be alive. All those years of physical and mental training helped Steve to survive and wake up from all those times he'd been in a diabetic coma and did not know it.

After getting much needed pills to regulate his blood sugar, Steve started training again. He began training with isometrics exclusively and used whatever he could get a hold of, like bike racks, playground equipment, cars, trucks, combines, trailers in various directions and positions – standing, kneeling, legs wide, etc. During this time he began to rebuild his body. The doctors had told him that he may never regain full use of his legs and feet. After a year and a half of isometric training, Steve was feeling better and getting pretty strong and was in fact able to do a feat he'd never been able to do even at his largest and strongest. For years he'd tried the lift the front wheel of a grain truck off the ground. A legendary feat he'd heard of, but had never seen done. Yet even after all the health problems and loss in size with the training he shows you in this book he was able to lift the truck wheel. Not bad for someone who wasn't able to walk!

After losing all his nerve sensation and power in his feet, Steve managed to regenerate those nerves through isometrics and controlling his blood sugar. He also began to take a few health supplements such as coral calcium, fish oil, olive oil, wheatgrass, MSM pills and seaweed. He believes these were very helpful in healing his nerves. This was enough for Steve to essentially cure his diabetes and recover fully. He doesn't take pills for diabetes anymore, as he believes they have very serious side effects.

His diet had to be changed completely as well. The first things he removed from his diet were beer and sodas, practically anything with lot of sugars and carbs. Steve also started eating 5 smaller meals per day instead of a couple of big ones. This resulted in faster metabolism, plus his pancreas wasn't overloaded on the insulin. The bigger your stomach is, the more insulin your body takes, which increases your chance to get diabetes.

Steve believes and has done a pretty good job of showing isometrics training will make you feel younger and working in many directions in various exercises will help you recover the nerves that get damaged over the years. Steve was actively involved in weight lifting, basketball, running, swimming and bicycling, but says nothing makes you feel as good as isometrics. His experience is that even if you get injured during other activities, isometrics will help you to get better through training of uninjured spots on your body. This will get your blood moving, activate your nerves, which will twitch in the injured area (despite the fact you are not training that specific area). Nerves are connected and act as units and can regrow in over-lapping patches where new nerves take over for old nerves. Steve believes this will help you heal up to ten times quicker! That's why he's decided to share his experience and this training with the world.

How I Got Started in Isometrics

I got interested in being strong when I saw a guy with huge arms at a rodeo when I was a kid. So I started to lift weights. Every once in a while I'd get hold of book or two and learn a few things. That's where I learned about power lifters and the old time strongmen. These guys were huge and strong and that's what I wanted to be. That's what I was getting until I had a problem.

You see I got this job working with a custom hay hauler. My boss owned the business and he was much older than me and in incredible shape. The thing is – I was stronger in many ways than him, but I couldn't keep up. He worked circles around me and laughed the whole time and that was a kick in the pride so to speak. Then one day I read a friend of mine's book on isometrics. These guys were doing isometrics on a power rack, (which is in a way more suitable for certain isometrics than what I showed you here, it is a different kind than I normally practice). The guy in the book was in incredible shape and very toned everywhere. That's the thing I came to realize with isometrics – It gives you a tougher look, opposite to weight lifting which usually revolves around muscle mass instead of definition. So it clicked with me that isometrics, training without actually moving, pushing against something that won't budge, might actually help me keep up with my crazy boss.

As the famous old time strongman Arthur Saxon said, "The more muscles you work, the better." With isometrics you can really work all those little muscles. Arthur used to work short pulls, heavy pulls, overloads, holds, one arm, two arm and even heavy singles on his bent press for hours. People said he was actually getting stronger at the end of his workout, since he knew how to pace himself. That's what I was missing. I wasn't getting all the little muscles and angles necessary to have coordinated strength to actually be able to use all that power I'd built with heavy weightlifting in the real world.

This happens all the time. Think of someone who is squatting tons of weight, but still manages to twist his ankle or get his knee ripped to pieces on a football field. It's because he is working his big muscles in up and down movements, but neglecting those small muscles, ligaments, joints and nerves which are weak and prone to injuries without isometrics training.

At my strongest days, I used to bench 475 pounds and sometimes I would punch those punching bag machines that test your power. There were many athletic guys who were hitting those bags much harder than I did even though I was stronger. That's because they were generating more power through their little muscles which gave them speed strength. That being said, isometrics are one of the best things any boxer, wrestler, MMA fighter, basketball player, football player should add to his training routine, because it can really give you speed and strength on the field or mat. For fighters especially, doing all isometrics along with punch training in different positions is what I'd recommend – up on their toes, wide, narrow, in squatted position and punches in all different directions.

So I start really hammering the isometrics and they helped me tremendously with the hay bales. I was finally getting the useable, coordinated, enduring strength that I wanted. One day we had to load around 300 bales and my boss and I made a deal to take our pulses before we started and once again five minutes after we were done. After we finished moving all those bales, it turns out his pulse was faster than mine. I was in that good of shape and I finally out-did him!

You can imitate any kind of movement with isometrics. For instance, if your goal is to do 1000 pushups, just place your hands on a bar simulating the push up position and push against it. Push in bursts, push hard, sometimes push and hold for time. Keep doing it for a couple of hours each day and in a few months the results will speak for themselves. Even though you can do just isometrics, if you are looking to improve your weight lifting or specific sport results, I recommend you combine them to get there much, much faster. Whatever you train for, be it bent press, handstand pushups or anything else, you need to actually work on that particular movement in order to get better at it. Isometrics are there to fill in the blank spots. For example, if you do a lot of isometrics and slack on weight lifting, you are obviously going to have a hard time achieving good results in weight lifting and vice versa. Isometrics can however stand completely alone and I believe that they will give you great all-around results even in things you don't train for.

Unfortunately as you've already read I didn't keep up with the conditioning and health that I build through my first experiments with isometrics, but I learned a ton and even though I nearly died, I was able to rebuild my health and strength at a much lighter bodyweight with this training.

Maybe one day you'll get crazy like me and really see how far you *can* go with isometrics. For a while to make all these exercises a bit tougher, I trained with a 300 pound chain-vest I made. I worked up to an hour straight using different pulling, pushing and twisting motions. That was really intense and beneficial in terms of endurance and you can really go places you never dreamed of when you train hard.

So I hope you're ready to train hard and learn a ton about isometrics.

Why Isometric Training is Effective, Beneficial and Efficient

A. The speed from which you can move from one exercise to another is great.
B. The number of angles and directions you can work exercises is almost unlimited
C. You can work multiple directions of force per exercise
D. Isometrics are great for rehabilitating injuries
E. Isometrics are great for body sculpting
F. Isometrics are great for strength or endurance training
G. Isometrics are great for working all your joints in a 360 angle to toughen joints, tendons and ligaments in all angles to toughen body to prevent injuries
H. Isometrics are great for building speed strength, holding strength and spot strength and toughness
I. Isometrics are fun and build your concentration mind, nerves, tendons and ligaments and muscle density
J. With isometrics it's easy to push or pull yourself at the rate that fits within your limits

Getting Started

When you start anything new start out slow and toughen in at a natural pace. Assess your physical state. Give your body at least a month to start adapting and toughening in. On movements you've done with weights, it's okay to go to a higher intensity faster. However when it comes to angles and positions you've never concentrated on before take it slow with less intensity till you toughen in. If you go all out on angles and positions you're not used to practicing chances are good you'll end up tearing something lose.

Everybody's body is different. Different bone thickness, different bone lengths, different degrees of nerve development in different areas. Lung development, endurance, strength, recuperation times are different, diet is different, the way you think is different. Your stress levels are different. So when you train your results will be different. And the amount of work you can do per session will be different. Learn to satisfy yourself, train at your own pace, experiment, never take anybody's word for anything at 100%. Learn to know yourself. Have your goals in your soul and have fun. Challenge yourself.

How To Gauge Your Progress

Depending on your goal:

1 For Strength

You'll learn to feel the power of your contraction, and how high a percentage of your maximum strength you're generating. The stronger you get in any exercise, the more power and harder contraction you'll generate in that exercise and outside in the real-world. You'll be able to feel it as you get stronger if you pay attention.

2 For Endurance

As you get in better shape the quicker you'll be able to go between exercises, or the more reps you'll be able to do or the more sets you'll be able to do, or the longer you'll be able to do holds without being overly tired.

3 For Strength, Speed, Endurance, The Overall

You'll be able to judge by how you feel, how you look, how you move and your lightness of foot. It's how fast you recuperate between workouts. The more advanced you become the less rest you'll need. If you want to be bigger, add more work at maximum intensity at squat, pull and press style moves. You want more endurance? Work more angles faster. If you want to bring a specific body part up, then work on longer holds and concentrate on that specific body part. If you want to be faster work on fast contractions at high intensity, then work on the move outside of isometrics that you actually want to be fast on.

Different Things to Use To Practice On

What I show in the book is just a very small number of things and exercises that can be done. It would take a book six inches thick to cover all the angles and objects you could use to train with. So it's important that you think for yourself, use your imagination and your mind to explore, but here are a few hints to help you.

Isometrics is technically pushing or pulling against things that don't move, but there is more to it. Isometrics is either for reps or holds. You can for example use our own body against itself, which is like the old time muscle control artists or the old time Charles Atlas courses. You can even do combinations of those styles where you are flexing a muscle or using the body against itself in combination with many other outside implements to push or pull against. You can even do an isometric contraction for one part of the body while moving other parts of the body.

You can use tables, chairs, benches, doorways, steel frames, hand rails, cars, trucks, heavy equipment, trees, telephone poles, pliers, bolts, power racks, bars, slings, frames that hold weights or machines, playground bars, or you can build your own equipment. Any kind of heavy steel, fire hydrants, walls, steps, anything you can push or pull against in any position will work. There's literally 1000's of things you can use to get a good workout on like car steering wheels, car dashes, heavy trailers, rocks, car floorboards for leg presses while using the seat to brace your back.

I can and have gotten a good workout in almost anywhere at any time. I've stood in bars and night clubs and taverns using my body against itself, or leaning on bar counters or chairs and all while people watching, but still training myself and nobody even knows it. I could get a great workout in a phone booth, or laying in bed watching TV.

Rep Training – High Reps / Medium Reps

One of my favorite ways to do isometrics is rep training. I've done anywhere from one rep to 10,000 reps. For example, I've done a quarter squat, standing position, 10,000 quick pushes with a bar behind my neck. I was probably using 25% of my maximum power output each surge, because I was working endurance. I kept this up for 50 minutes straight without a rest. When I hit 10,000 reps I got out from underneath that bar and my whole body felt like a rock.

You could do ten reps at 90% for 20 sets, or you can do 100 reps for 100 sets and you'll do your 100 reps at about 60% max. You could do 100 different exercises, three sets of five reps each and do your five reps at 75% power. I mean the possible combinations with reps and sets with these isometrics are virtually endless and I've done them all, because I like all around training.

I've also done 1,000 different exercises per workout, one rep each at 100% max. I really like this one because it builds all-around endurance, strength and speed. It's fun to experiment. When I train I have no set routine, no set exercises, no set number of reps, sets or holds. There are no set times or days. I do everything on the mood I'm in and the spur of the moment challenge, but that's just me. Everybody needs to do things their own way. If you feel like you need a regular routine, pick one of the ways I've listed above and write down the individual exercises that are important to you and do that once or twice a week, until you feel you've really gained power in those specific movements. On the other days I still suggest you learn to go with your intuition, because you're body will tell you what it needs to get to your goals if you listen.

Remember that all this training is flowing to the same point of greater strength anyway – so even if you vary from day to day, so long as you're circling towards the goal you want and working hard, you'll get there.

Training For Maximum Strength

First figure out what exercises you want to get strong in then this is what I'd do:

I'd do three sets and this is what I describe as a set. For example top dead lift position or ¼ deadlift bar is just about 3" above the knees. This is one continuous movement or effort. Pull, lock and hold, relax just a tad. Take another breath and hold breath, then pull a little harder, lock and hold. Then relax just a little tiny bit, take another breath and hold, then pull, lock and hold harder, then repeat till you've done this four times and each time you try to dig deeper and pull harder. You're locking and loading a little harder each time till the fourth effort is your total maximum pull.

I call this the Four Serge Technique. It teaches you to dig way down deep inside yourself. You're generating maximum nerve power. I call this one set. The four surges is one set then do these four surges three different times and then we'll call this three sets.

Say you want to use this for this example to improve your deadlift. Do three sets in five positions of the surge sets:

3 surge sets bottom
3 surge sets mid shin
3 surge sets at knee height
3 surge sets at mid thigh
3 surge sets at very top

This is the example for the deadlift.

As one example this type of training develops maximum pulling or pushing power and can be applied to any exercises or combination of exercises you want to get strong in. This type of training will wear you out fast, but will give you the maximum strength in the things you want to get the strongest in. I would recommend when you go all out like this to do this every other day. And if you prefer, on the days in between, you can fill in by doing other exercises at a lower intensity. Again the combinations are endless.

If you chose to get strong or get maximum strong in just three or four exercises, this type of training will produce maximum strength effect. This also teaches you how to unleash your nerve power to the max. Now as to how many exercises you want to do this way is your call and you'll have to figure that out for yourself, because everybody is at a different endurance and toughness. Learn to feel how much you can take or how hard you can push yourself. I am going to suggest, however, that you start with five positions and three sets each on a squat, a press, a pull and then an arm and abdominal movement. If you feel like you can do more, you can add to it, but I would concentrate on them and be sure

I was working at maximum intensity before I added more volume. You can test this by working in other actual lifting movements you want to get strong in, just to see how it's working. Also if you want to get strong at some specific move that doesn't fit what I've already listed, like say punching, or lifting some object for strongman training or tackling for football or grappling, then simply break down the movement the same way and apply that same movement directly to the thing you want to get strong at.

Another great way is to do squats, presses and pulls every other day and on your off days do the specific move that is out of the ordinary or non-linear that you want to get strong in along with whatever else you feel like doing that day.

Jerk or G-Force Reps

Now and then I do what I call Jerk or G-Force reps which I use about a ¼ inch of play on the isometric pushing or pulling and I use an explosion of power to a sudden stop.

The sudden stop is what toughens you up. You can do this in many of exercises or just a few, it's up to you. Be careful though you have to be pretty toughened in for this type of training.

A good example for this is get on a hard floor in your socks or bare feet, raise up on your toes, lock all your joints solid and drop straight down on your heels. That sudden stop with everything locked solid will send a shock wave through your whole body. This type of training is good for toughening bone density. Its kind of like training to break things in karate breaking. It's like beating your fists on a brick wall or kicking a tree or smashing your shoulder into a brick wall or stomp-walking.

I also use this with the specialty isometric rack I have or the classic isometric rack that I use by literally grabbing and doing a pushing and pulling movement against the rack super fast. It's great for building speed and reversing direction. Even if the rack doesn't move, I'm attempting to "jerk it," back and forth and make it move each direction. You can do very high intensity with this and very high reps, very fast. You can also go directly from longer holds to jerk-reps to switch back and forth.

Holding for Time

Doing Isometrics holding for time builds great endurance and great strength and is truly a challenge and a lot of fun.

Pick your exercises that you want to do this way then pick your time in your mind that you're going to hold the hold for. Of course the longer you hold or pull or push the less intensity you'll have to use. I've done up to 10 minute holds in certain things. Let me tell you this kind of training really builds mental toughness and will give you some really sore muscles and tendons if you're not used to it. Every now and again I will do some of this type of training.

Another way to do this while you're building up to an advanced style of training or sometimes to even make advanced training more difficult is to use surges within the time holds. For instance when you're starting you might be trying to hold five minutes at 50% at a particular push or pull or position. You can add small bursts of say 70% of more during that five minutes to get more strength while you're building up or if you're really having trouble you might drop to say 40% pressure as long as you don't give up on the push or pull. When you've recovered a little bit go right back to 50%. When you're advanced you might be trying to hold 10 minutes at 60%,and to make it harder you could do bursts of 80-90%, maybe dropping back to 60%, but never leaving the push or pull for the amount of time you've chosen to hold.

I've done several workouts where I held a particular isometric for three minutes, rested one minute and repeated five to ten times. I also did a hold of 10 minutes each in six different exercises to make a full hour holding. The possibilities here are endless.

Angles and Positions

What a lot of people don't realize is that there are infinite training positions of the body. Each position determines what different nerves, muscles and tendons and ligaments get worked. There are over 600 different muscles in the body so you can only imagine how many different combinations of interaction are going to have to go on to stimulate all these different nerves' angles.

You have flat footed, on toes, legs close, legs wide, legs split, legs full squat, half squat, waist sideways, waist bent over, waist straight, waist bent backwards, neck twist, neck bend forward, back and sideways, leg twist, hip rotation front, sideways and back. Arm and wrist twist, overhead side, down, arm straight, arm bent, finger pulls, twists – You start throwing all these combinations together it will add up to thousands of different disciplines of exercises. Just use your imagination. Every different position you're in performing an exercise pulls different nerves and muscles in to play from different angles and also gives you more endurance and more coordination.

What I believe sets my isometrics apart from those other people have experimented with is the fact that I try to add multiple combinations of these basics together at the same time. For instance in much of the training you'll see in the pictures in this book, I am pushing or pulling literally in multiple directions at the same time. If you think about it the work you do in real life usually isn't just a straight angle. It's lifting a thing, pushing or pulling it away from yourself and then moving with it often while you twist. That is three to four different directions of pressure at the same time. Certainly you should do some high percentage of strength moves, where you push in a simple one direction angle. You should also think through the moves you're doing into the multiple directions you could be pushing or pulling with each move. For example in a squat, deadlift or press type move you can obviously push or pull just straight up and down, but you can also push or pull up or down while simultaneously pushing forward or backward or while also twisting in or out and to the side. Those are basic variations of angles you can use to make this training crank up lots of little nerves and muscle you're probably not using on a regular basis. That is the key to making you super strong with this isometric training.

Philosophy of Nerve Power

Nerve power is something the old time strongmen talked about a great deal. When they said it they really meant the same thing as many of the eastern philosophies mean when they talk about "Chi." It is a combination of the actual nerves that run through your muscles and make things happen when your mind tells the body to move and the subtle electrical current that flows around the whole body that actually makes those nerves function. Isometrics are proven to be one of the greatest ways to turn your nerves on or bring them up to their highest potential and therefore bring your muscle's ability to contract up to its greatest strength.

My thinking on nerve power is that building your nerve power or endurance is the true secret of really getting to be a super athlete. When you train you not only build your body strength, your tendons, ligaments and muscles, but also your nerve power. So when you're trained all around from all angles you train your nerves and all their crossing routes and the more angles you train the more developed your nerve highways will be and the better your endurance will be all around.

Because the truth is if you exhaust one little nerve to failure it can virtually tire your whole body out. I believe the more nerves you bring in to play in training the better overall health you'll have and the better your energy will flow from one part of your body to another and the more coordinated you'll be and the more stamina you'll have.

In my opinion the better you train your nerves the faster your body recuperates and the less sleep you actually need.

Building Energy Through Isometrics

Isometrics work a wide range of muscles, nerves and angles at the same time. The problem is that little muscles are generally weak point for most people, both in terms of strength and energy, and if you manage to improve those weak spots, your whole body energy will improve.

Most people take tons of protein in their diet and do 5 reps in first set, four in the second set and down to sets of 3,2 and 1 reps. Their energy comes from the food, but from my point of view the energy is built through more sets, more work, different exercises and their variations, longer holds and increased intensity. This way you'll build your bodily energy without an excess intake of food.

Use your will power instead of steroids. Likewise, use your bodily energy to train more and more to become stronger. For example, a person who is able to run fifty miles didn't start out with that distance, but gradually increased it over time through regular training and energy building.

Using this technique you don't need to take a bunch of protein powder every day. That's what I used to do when I was a kid and it actually ruined my health. With isometrics, you are slowly increasing your strength, energy, nerve power and endurance.

Basically, what you want is to turn yourself into more powerful and efficient machine which doesn't need as much fuel. The energy in the muscle itself becomes higher, so you don't need as much energy in a form of food to keep progressing.

People who do isometrics regularly become stronger the longer and harder they push. The reason for this is that they aren't burning energy up while pushing, but they are creating energy as they go.

Through isometrics training, you are basically building your bodily energy and training your nerves. When you twitch them, they activate and receive oxygen and nutrients, which makes them stronger. As your nerves become stronger and stronger, so will your muscles, since you can contract them stronger. Just pace yourself and train slowly to make a gradual progress. You don't need to eat tons of steaks and eggs, just eat normal and use your will power instead to do more work and build physical power.

For maximum power training, I would recommend training only once or twice a week, hour and a half each session. If you are already in a good shape, training isometrics several hours after the weight training is also a good idea.

For maximum endurance, I'd recommend doing a wide range of exercises and mix everything as much as possible with long holds, high reps with many different directional movements. It would be great if you could do every joint in a circle, to cover movements in all directions.

Training the Mind

Your mind is the best weapon you have in the battle for super strength or super endurance or both. When you train the body, you also train your mind and your will power. The more and longer you train the more you train your mind. The hardest thing in the world for most people is to change their body especially to gain super strength and endurance.

Some of the old time strong men like Saxon and Cyr and Anderson talked about the more your train the more psychic or intuitive you'll become, because you learn how to connect your conscious mind with your subconscious mind, you'll start to bridge the gap. When you work a normal exercise until you can do it without thinking and apply your whole being to it, this is what you're doing. Isometrics make this even simpler, because they are so simple in themselves. You can then apply what you are consciously thinking with the effort of your whole being connecting the two for greater mind and body power.

If you can see things in your mind long enough and hard enough your mind will figure out a way to make it happen. What you see and think about creates its own momentum and eventually materializes into reality so build your will power by training hard and long or just enough each time to make you satisfied with yourself. Whatever you think about the most and hardest will create the power for you if you so desire. Your mind will show you the way to make the unbelievable, believable.

My theory On Sports Injuries

My theory on a lot of sports injuries is basically most people over work the big muscles and neglect the small ones. Then when force is applied to areas that aren't toughened in, something tears loose. This is why every joint should be worked in 360 degrees from all angles. In my opinion this would prevent a whole lot of these sports injuries from occurring. And isometrics are a great way to do this safely.

This is especially applicable for the ankles, knees and shoulders, but could be applied to any joint. We almost always train in a very straight up and down fashion in normal weightlifting, yet on the ball field or court we subject ourselves to courses that are not straight at all. Every time a football or basketball player steps to the side he's creating lateral torque on all his joints, not just straight up and down torque like most weight lifting. So why don't we train that? Because it's very hard to do with a barbell or machine. If you're rehabilitating one of these injuries or simply training to make those moves as fast and safe as possible, or make those joints as resistant to injury as possible then I suggest you train those joints with lateral pushing and pulling movements. It's simple to do and can build muscles you can hit any other way, therefore making you safer and stronger or faster.

Combining Isometrics with other Forms of Training

Now to be the best or at the top of your game in any discipline, you have to practice that exact discipline. It is a matter of nerve coordination and feel. In my opinion isometrics is a way to give you a great all around strength that could be integrated to fit or compliment anything you are trying to be good at - Any other type of lifting, training, or sport or daily job. If you want to be all around tougher and better conditioned I would add at least a couple hours a week of isometric training to your arsenal. What you do or how you do it is up to you, you'll have to figure that out for yourself.

Obviously, the beauty of isometrics is that you can copy any position that you can't do with normal weight lifting. Therefore you can get strong at things that just don't quite carry over from lifting a bar. Most of you have probably read the story from my first book, Rock, Iron, Steel, about me working for a custom hay hauling business. How I was light years stronger than the guy I worked with, but he'd work circles around me because he was very used to the specific physical ability and I wasn't. The question is, how do you get used to a physical ability that doesn't have a set pattern? The answer is isometrics. When I added them in many different angles, I suddenly was able to keep up and apply strength in many different ways I'd never been able to do before. It took my normal weightlifter strength and turned it into all around strength, because I was using angles and getting used to the body using nerve patterns, making one strength flow to another.

If you're going to use Isometrics for adding to your normal muscle building, I suggest you switch them out every other session. One session with normal weights or lifts or whatever you're training – the next with isometrics for all-around or the thing you specifically want to get strong at. Use common sense here. If you want to get strong use higher percentage of maximum isometrics. However test it and see how it effects you because it is an individual thing. Realize that isometrics is very dense training. A ten second absolute maximum hold is like doing many reps at a very high intensity. Therefore it can be easy to burn out if you're working too hard in combining it with normal weights or strongman training. Try one or two max sets and see how it affects you the next time you do heavy lifting. Then you can modify to get the best result. Remember your nerves need to rest and recuperate just like anything else and that's really what you're training with isometrics. Also to get the best result you want to do isometrics in you strongest position and your weakest position. That way you actually get stronger where you need it and you open up the nerves for higher strength where you'll actually already strong.

Routines I've done Myself

When it comes to isometrics I've done about every routine you could actually dream up.

Examples: Sometimes I'll do just one exercise for two hours straight, doing set after set after set, sometimes using high reps with less intensity, sometimes using low reps with high intensity, sometimes using minute long holds, sometimes using long 5 minute holds.

Sometimes I'll do 1,000 different exercises in a couple hours, one 10 second hold each exercise or one second burst. Sometimes I'll do 20 different things 3 sets of surges to maximum intensity, each exercise. The combinations are endless. Believe me I've done it all and for me it's whatever mood I'm in. There's nothing set in stone for me, I just like training. I will say the best shape I've ever been in was when I was training isometrics three to four hours a day seven days a week for six months straight. My endurance was phenomenal I had every little muscle and tendon cut and ripped. But for pure strength I would keep your training to not over 3 hours a week, five at the most.

I used to walk into bars wearing a tank top and everybody's head would turn because of the superior build I had. See when you're really toughened in it's a sight that is majestic and to really toughen in to get that magical look you have to do hundreds of different exercises. All the time. It's just a matter of what you want.

A couple of the pictures on the cover of my book are from when I trained for four hours a day, seven days a week for over six months straight. You should be able to see what I'm talking about. I was actually in far better condition than a tri-athlete would be.

Now if you're going for pure unadulterated strength I wouldn't go over five hours a week maybe three and half sessions. For me, I had far more fun being in super condition where I had every little muscle toned in than I had with the super strength on the heavy iron. It's all about priorities on what you want. Now what's nice is if you have a little bit of everything: super strength, super conditioning and endurance and super speed and coordination – that's the ultimate. Of course that's the hardest to obtain because it takes a lot of work and a longer time. When I was in that magical build state I would do 20,000 to 30,000 pushes and pulls of split-second bursts for 100 reps at a shot, each exercise and I'd move from one exercise to the next with no rest in between at all.

That's how good of condition I was in. A real good workout that I used to do was I'd pick out 100 different exercises or positions and do a seven second hold or push on each one going from one to another without any rest in between. Do this every other day this will give you great strength and a well rounded build.

Supplements I Use

The supplements I use are pretty basic. I've never used steroids and I don't take supplements steady. The way I do it is this:

First, the things I've relied on or use off and on are:

Multi-vitamin
Vitamin C
Vitamin E
Fish Oil (Omega 3)
Olive Oil
Wheat Grass
Kelp
MSM – A sulfur pill
B Vitamins
Coral Calcium

These are my basics. Sometimes I'll pop two or three of this or that, but nothing too steady. Just now and then and as far as food goes I just eat whatever is available or whatever I have a craving for.

Exercises On my Specialty Isometric Rack

The following pages and pictures will be just a few of the exercises you can do on my specialty isometric rack. I put this together to give many different angles and positions to pull from and to be able to move from exercise to exercise with little ro no rest because the handles are pre-set. Remember, you don't necessarily have to have a rack like this to do this work. Anything that won't move when you push or pull on it, that simulates the angles or positions I'm about to show you, will work. If you're interested in the plans for a rack like this, send us an email.

Quarter or Top-End Deadlift Isometrics

This is one of my favorites that I come back to all the time. It, and the quarter squat isometric, are two of my power moves, because you can generate a great deal of force and they make you very strong. This is perfect for the "Surge and Hold," technique for max tension explained earlier.

Grab the bar that is approximately 3" or so about the knees and pull on it as if attempting to straighten your body completely out. Set your feet in a solid position and get a good grip. Remember to breathe the right way for what you're specifically doing. You're going to hold and push the air out slowly for a max effort and breathe deeper and normally for a long hold. You can emphasize different muscles by putting your knees slightly under the bar, which works more of your legs or bending more at the waist which will work more of your back. You can also change your foot positions from close, to wide, closer or further from the bar, or stagger one foot in front of the other. I also like to do this by not just pulling straight up, but by adding multiple directions. For instance pulling up and twisting left or right, front or back and side to side.

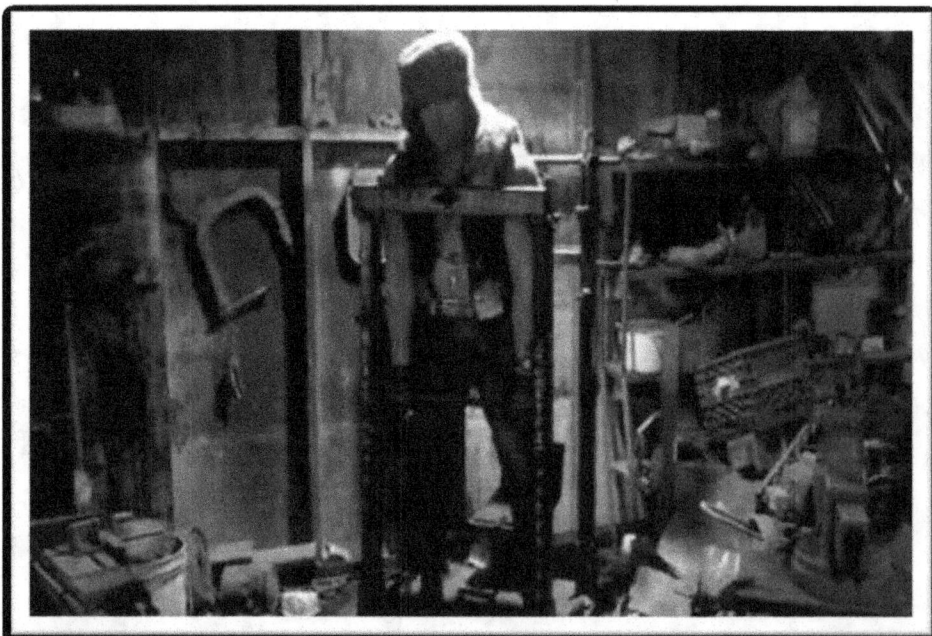

Quarter Deadlift with Multiple Direction Pressure

You can see in this picture I'm performing the quarter deadlift isometric, but I am leaning in to the rack so that I can add multiple directions of pressure with the rest of my body. Below are listed several variations.

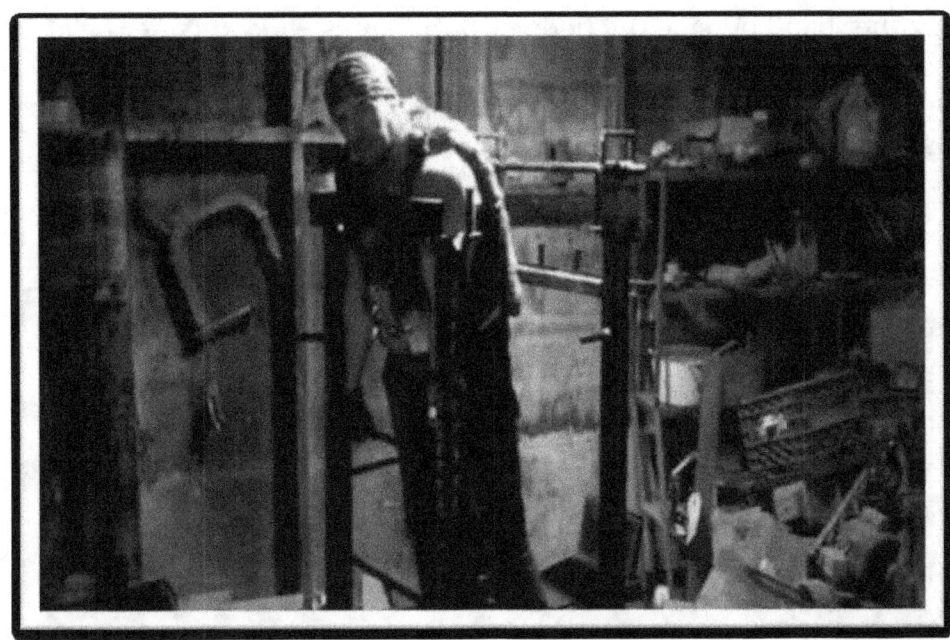

Variation 1: Quarter deadlift with front pressure into rack with chest and shoulders

Variation 2: Quarter deadlift with side pressure left or right with hands or chest and shoulders

Variation 3: Quarter deadlift with arms and shoulders pushing out against the rack at the same time.

Variation 4: Quarter deadlift with opposing pressure. One arm pulls up, the other pushes down.

Variation 5: Quarter deadlift with wrist twisting pressure.

Variation 6: Quarter deadlift while simultaneously trying to front-raise the bar

Variation 7: Quarter deadlift pulling up with both hands while twisting in and out

Variation 8: Push down with both hands and arms, while twisting your wrist in and out

Quarter Deadlift with Grip Variation

Shown here is the quarter deadlift done with hands together gripping to the left of the body. By shifting the pressure outside, your work the inside and outside thigh very hard. You can do this with knuckles facing forward or a curl grip or a split grip. Other variations include hands close or touching in the middle of the body, one hand in the of the body, the other hand outside the body or both hands wide outside the body. All of these can also be used with the other directional pressure variations such as forward, backward, wrist twist, one hand up, one hand down, etc. They can also be varied by foot stance or close, wide, staggered or on toes.

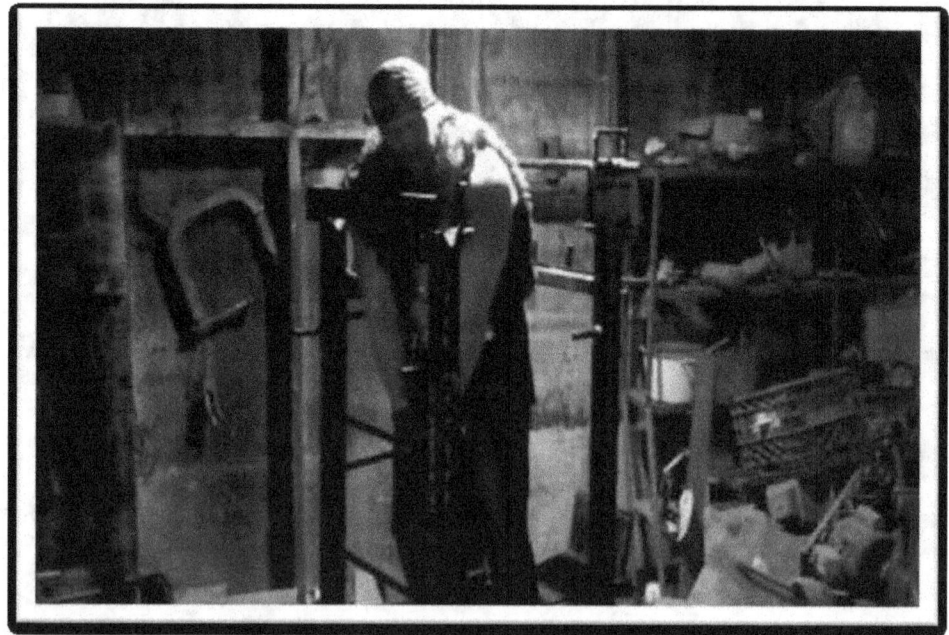

One-Handed Straight Outside Body Pull

This is pull is similar to the quarter deadlift, but done outside the body. You can alter it by standing closer or further away from the handle or using a straight or staggered stance. This series is perfect for Jerk Reps, which is how I often train this move. You can pull up and immediately push back down going very fast, creating a split-second isometric each way. You can also hold for different times, one second to one minute, each direction.

The next several pictures will show clear variations for adding multiple directions on top of the basic up and down pull. We won't show this for every isometric because it would literally be thousands of pictures, but on this one you can clearly see the multiple directions you can go at one time which adds to the effectiveness of the training.

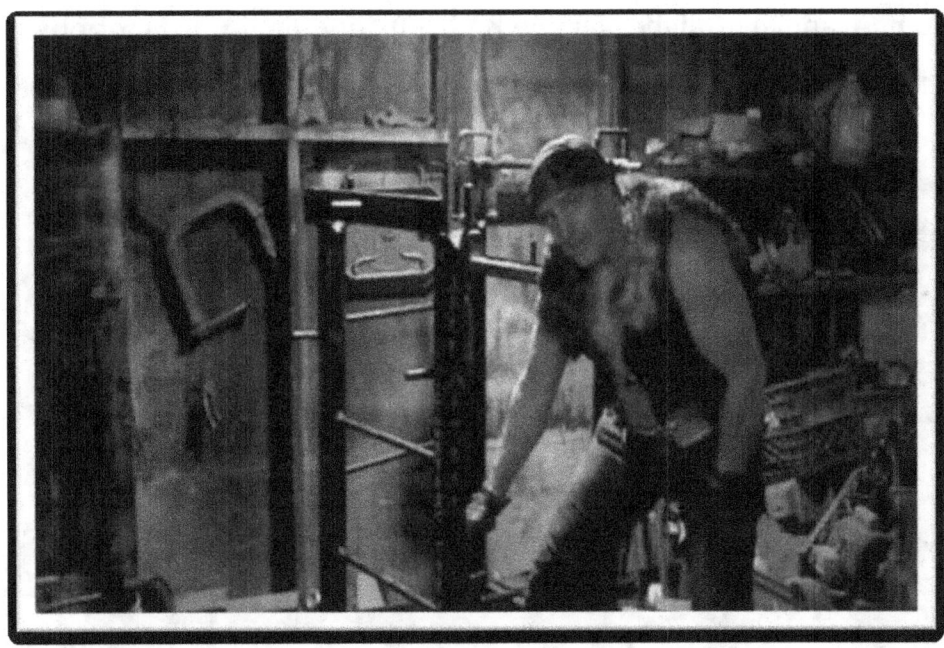

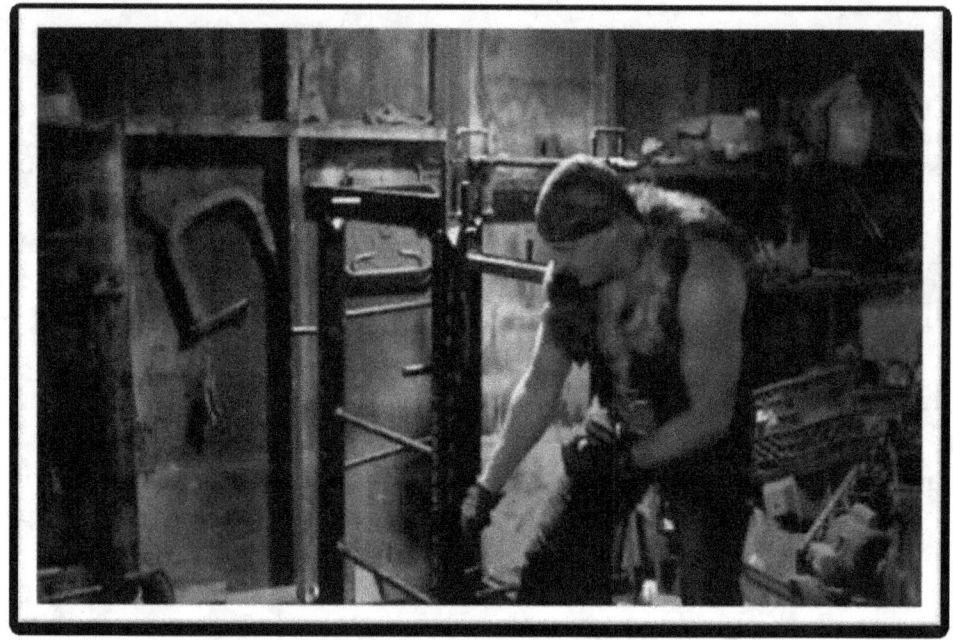

Variation 2: One-Handed Straight Outside Body Pull adding inward motion or pressure.

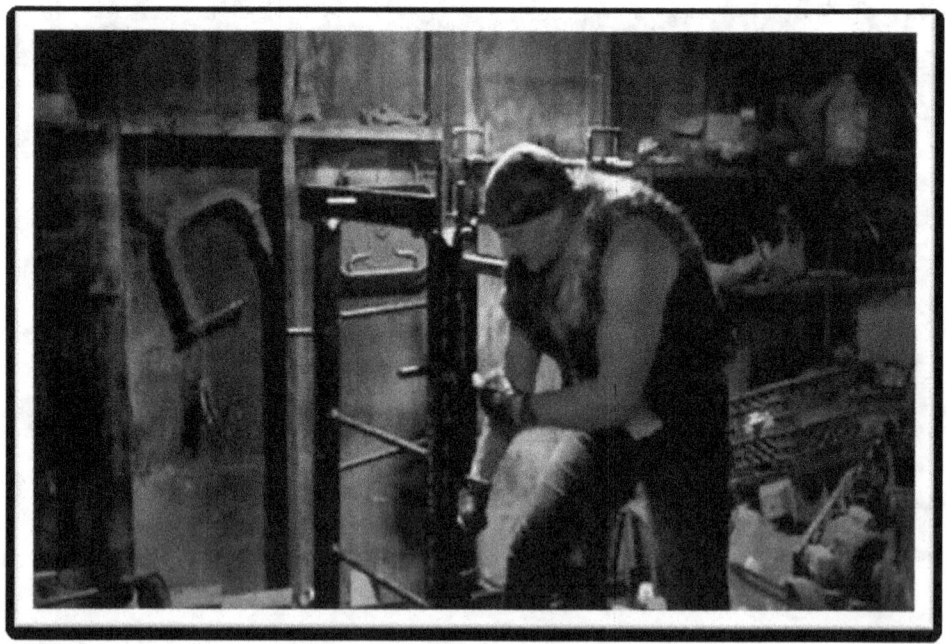

Variation 3: One-Handed Straight Outside Body Pull adding forward motion or pressure

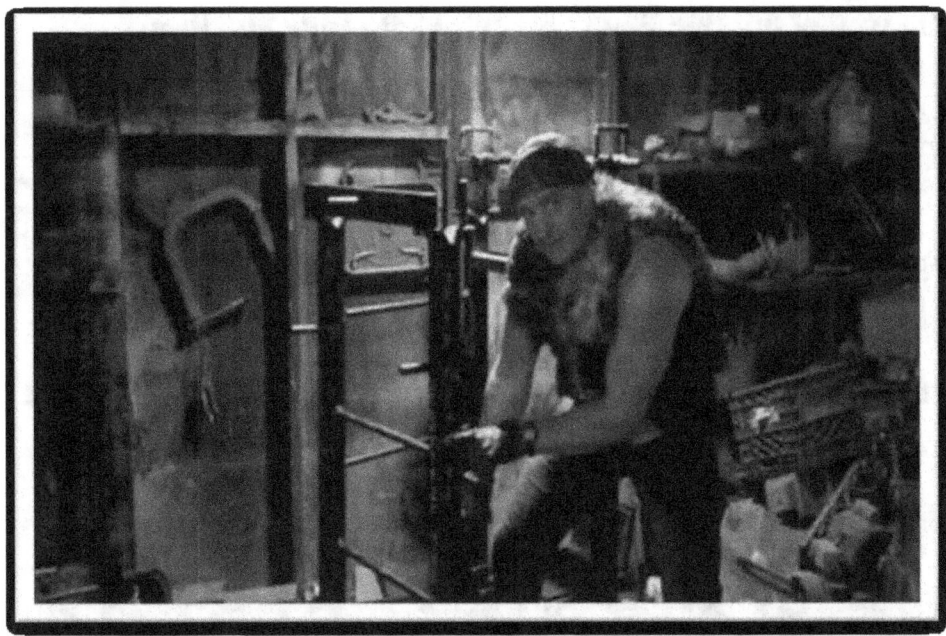

Variation 3: One-Handed Straight Outside Body Pull adding backward motion or pressure

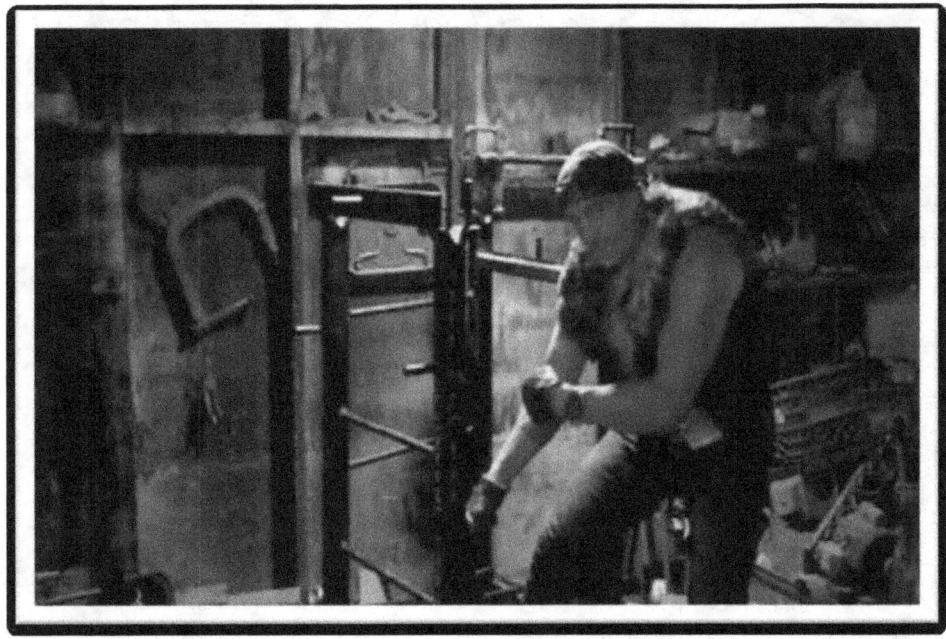

Variation 5: One-Handed Straight Outside Body Pull adding circular motion or pressure. This really works a lot of different muscles.

One-Handed Straight Outside Body Pull done with Lock and Hold

Another example of this, but using the, "Lock and Hold," method instead of Jerk Reps. Assume the same position as if you were to do jerks, but instead lock and hold with a straight back. Keep in mind you have to lock your whole body, no matter which isometric exercise you do.

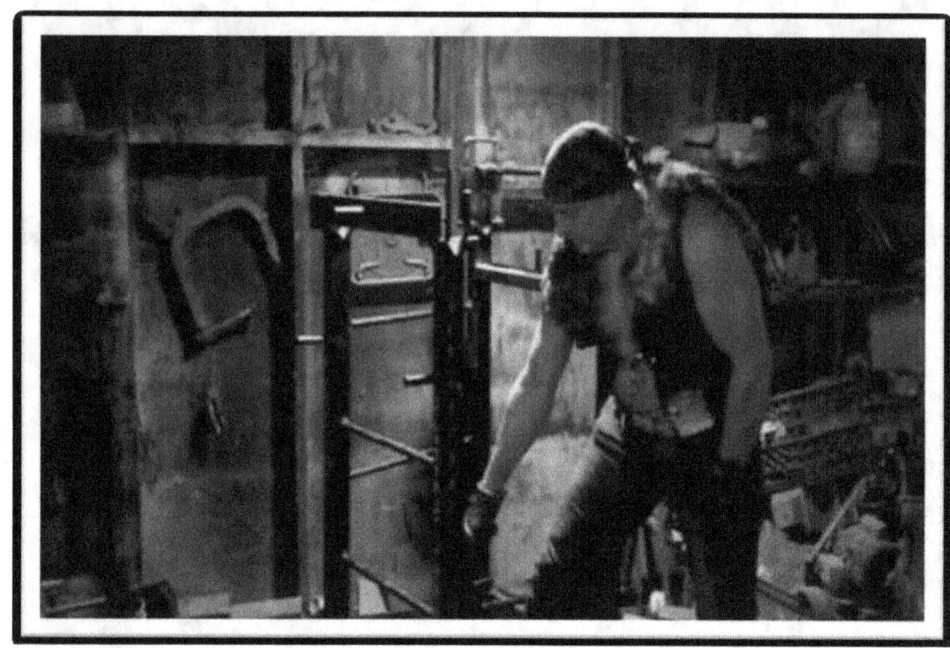

Variation 1: Lock and hold while pulling in

Variation 2: Lock and hold while pulling out

Variation 3: Lock and hold while pulling back

Variation 4: Lock and hold while pushing forward

Variation 5: Lock and hold pulling up/down and twist your wrist at the same time

Variations 6, 7 and 8: Lock and hold pulling in or out or forward or back AND adding a twist of your wrist in other directions

Down-push Arm Outside Body

Place one hand on the middle bar and the other one on top of the machine, like in the picture below.

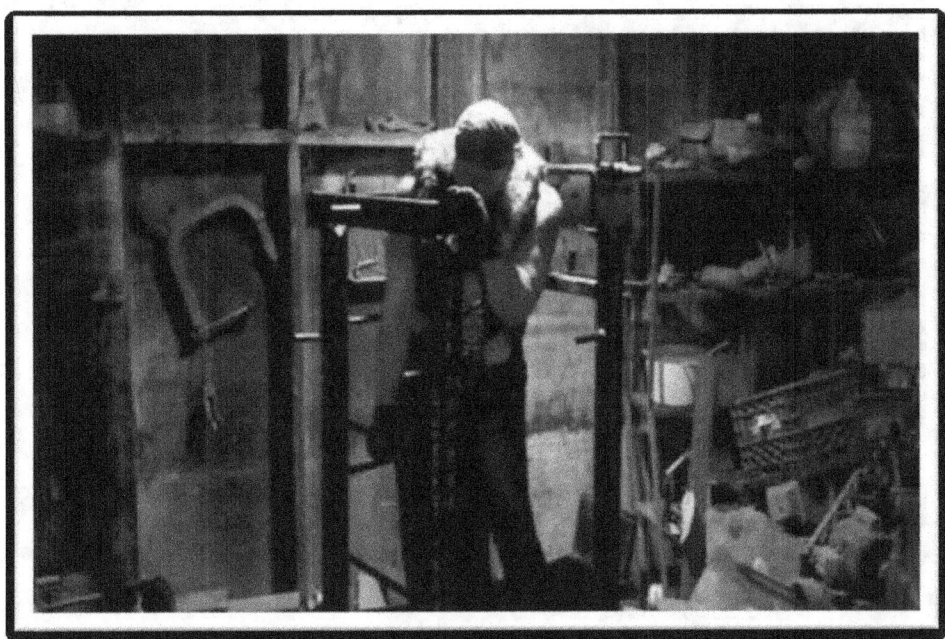

Variation 1: Anchor the body with the off-hand as shown in the picture and push straight down.

Variation 2: Push straight down and add back pressure trying to bring the arm behind the body.

Variation 3: Push straight down and add forward pressure trying to bring the arm to the front of the body.

Variation 4: Push straight down and try to twist the wrist forward or back or up and down.

Variation 5: Push straight down and add pressure straight to the side like a lateral raise or straight in front of the body pulling inward.

Variation 6: Push down at a 45 degree angle forward or backward of the body

Variation 7: Add any of the wrist twists or lateral motions to the 45 degree down push.

Pull Up and Pull Out While Holding Two Different Bars/Handles

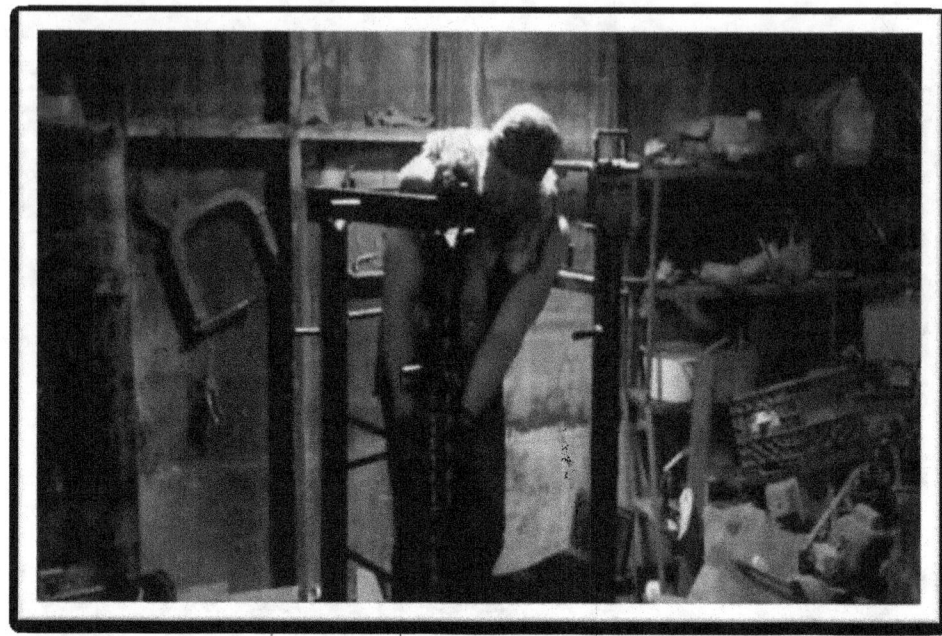

Variation 1: Place one hand on the middle bar, the other one on the handle (or another bar close to it, preferably at a slightly different angle, this will depend on what implement you're using to do this), and pull up and out at the same time, as if you were to rip the bar/handle apart.

Variation 2: Push your arms together at the same time while you are pulling up

Variation 3: Twist your wrists in while you are pulling and pushing your arms in

Variation 4: Twist your wrists out while you are pulling and pushing your arms in

Variation 5: Pull back with both of your arms to try and hit the muscles on the side of your abdomen

Variation 6: To hit a lot of muscles quickly, shift your pulls to the right, left and down sequentially.

Use your imagination for more variations. Pull in all directions until you are tired or just pull in and stay in that position for some time, twisting your wrist. You can also just grab the bar with both arms and go up and down, so you are basically pulling up and pushing down continuously in a rapid manner or doing Jerk Reps.

Reach Over Multi-Direction Pulls

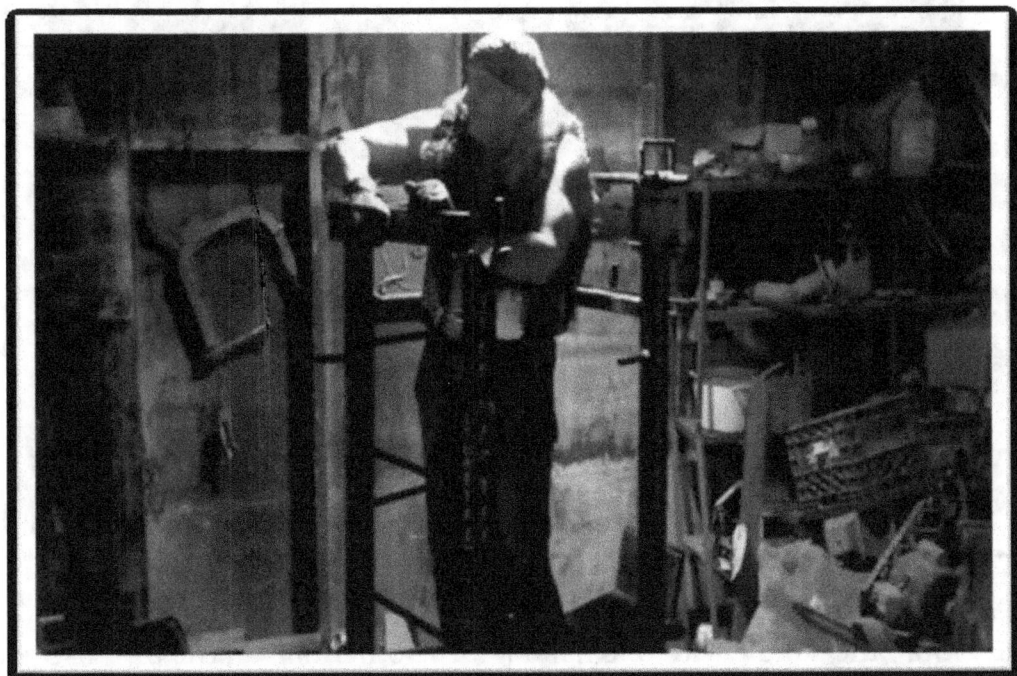

Variation 1: You can see this is similar to a working situation that any blue-collar guy might find himself in. Reach over the top of the frame, grab the upper handle and pull up and back while pushing the bar forward with your left hand. This is also great for grapplers as it simulates some of the positions you could be in with your hands locked while wrestling.

Variation 2: Pull up, back and in with your right or left hand.

Variation 3: Pull up, back, and out with right or left hand.

Variation 4: Grab the handles in the same position, but exaggerate your front, back or both arms higher or lower to create a different, more stretched position.

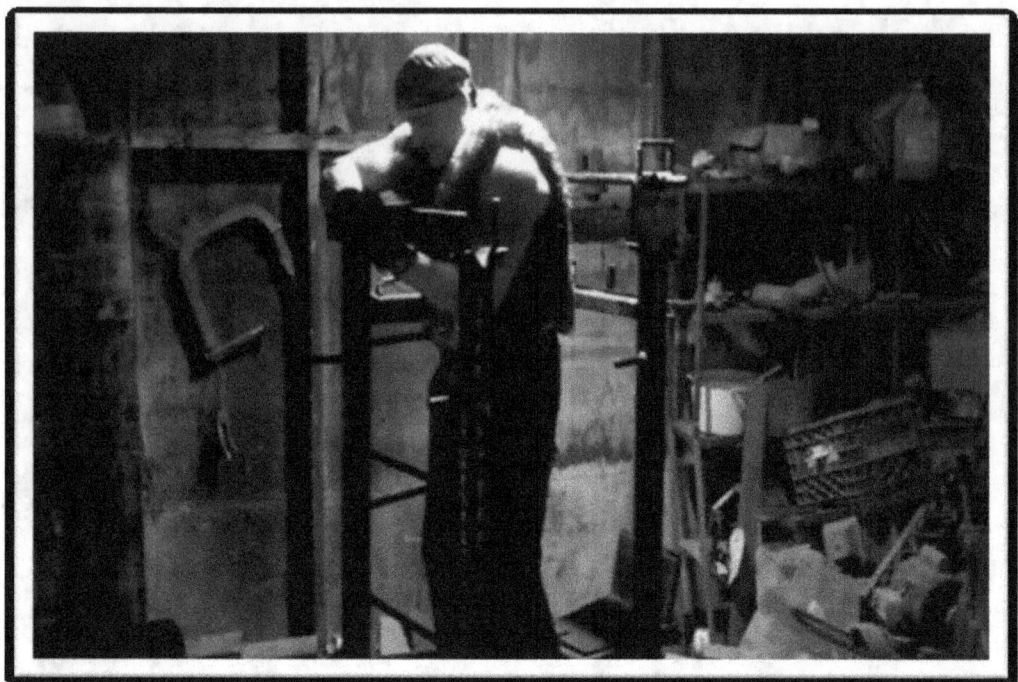

Variation 5: Grab the handle with one hand put the other one on the top. Use your whole body to move left and right. This one should really hit your twisting muscles in your legs. Possible variations of this variation include going up, down or out.

Grab and Twist

Grab the handle firmly and twist your wrist around in circles while you are pulling up or twist your wrist back and forth while you are pushing down. This one works many muscles at the same time. You can do this by twisting with the arms as well, pushing and pulling different directions with arms bent or arms straight or slowly or straightening and bending the arms as you concentrate on the wrists or torso. You can also lock the arms, then grab and twist using just your body (your arms transfer the power but don't move), using your side, leg and abdominal muscles and for ever more variation, grab a bar of different heights and do the same twists with the wrists or body.

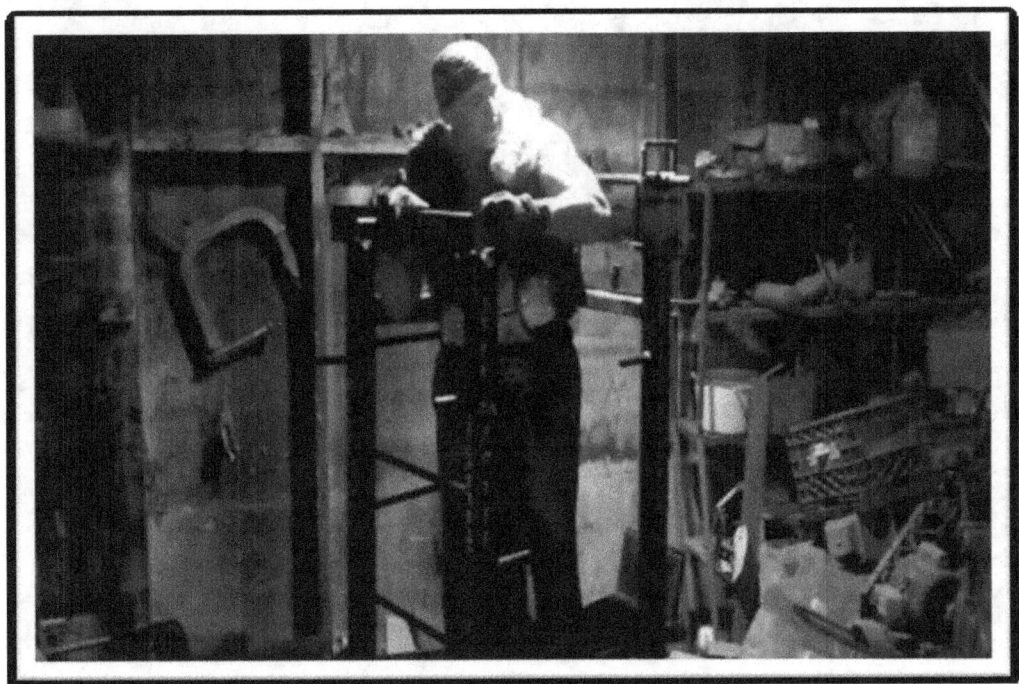

Isometrics for Running

Put your leg behind the frame bar and lock it using one of the handles, push it forward while pulling your other leg. Place your hands on top handles and pull back and forward in twisting motion, to imitate actual running motion. The pictures show one position and what would be a relatively short stride, but you can also use a much longer split-leg position, or multiple positions. You can also use the bar to block the knee to work on driving the knee forward instead of lifting the foot. Or simultaneously push off the back foot and forward with the knee at the same time.

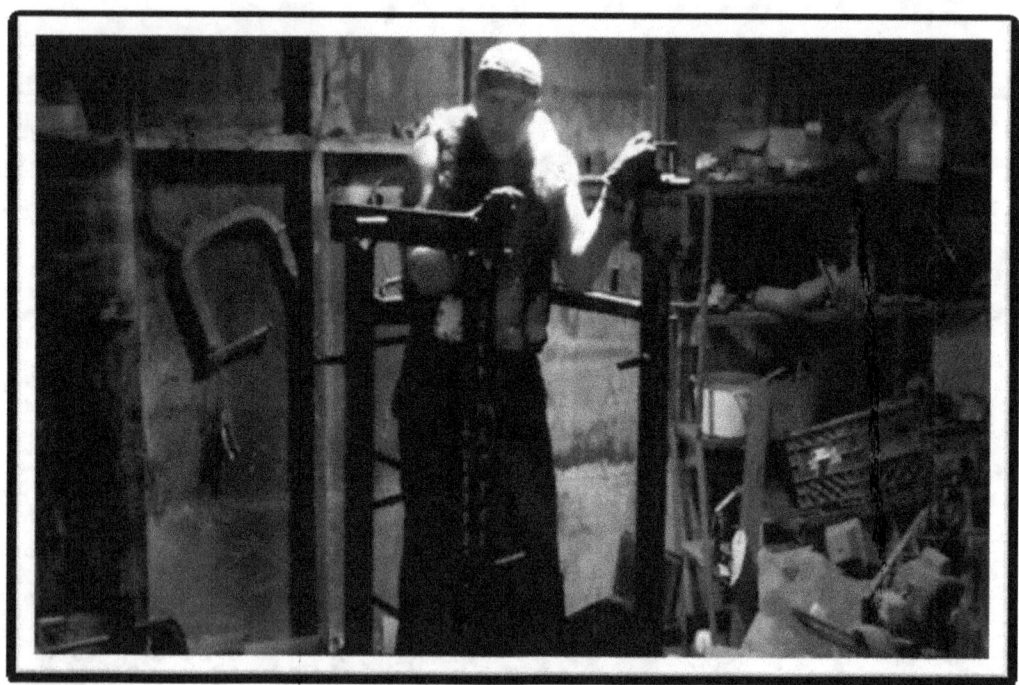

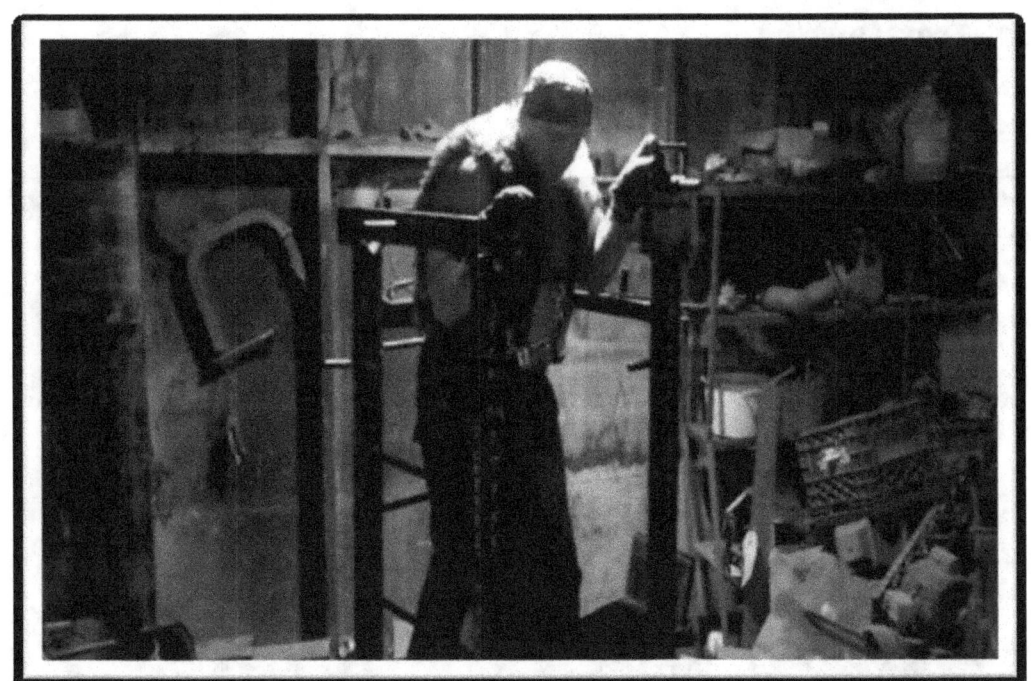

Pull Up and Twist Legs

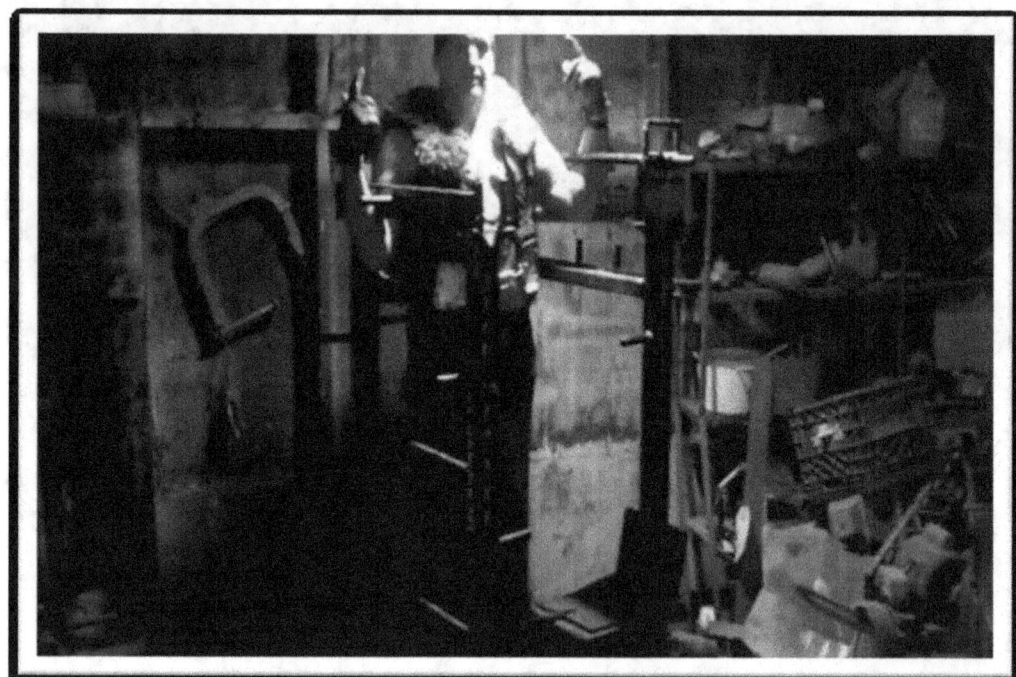

Variation 1: Lock your arms beneath the bars and pull them up while putting pressure on your legs and twisting them in. Heels in, heels out. This is similar to a Zercher lift where the bar is in the crook of your arms, but in my rack your arms are pointing directly out instead of forward.

Variation 2: Let your arms down and get up on your toes. Push your legs forward, pull them backward, go in and out.

Variation 3: Hook just one arm under the bar and use your body to make the up, in, back and twisting motions.

Variation 4: Hook both arms under the bar and stand on one leg and repeat the squat, up, in, out and twisting motion.

Variation 5: Same motion, but hook one arm under the bars and stand on one leg. These can be same side or opposite side. i.e., hook with right arm, stand on right leg, hook with right arm, stand on left leg.

Variation 6: Use the same elbow hooking motion, but on a lower set of bars so you're in a deeper squat or lunge position and repeat the up, in, out and twist.

Variation 7: Hook your arms on uneven bars, one higher or lower and repeat the motions. Or put a block under one foot so that it's higher than the other and repeat the same motions.

Quarter Squat Isometric

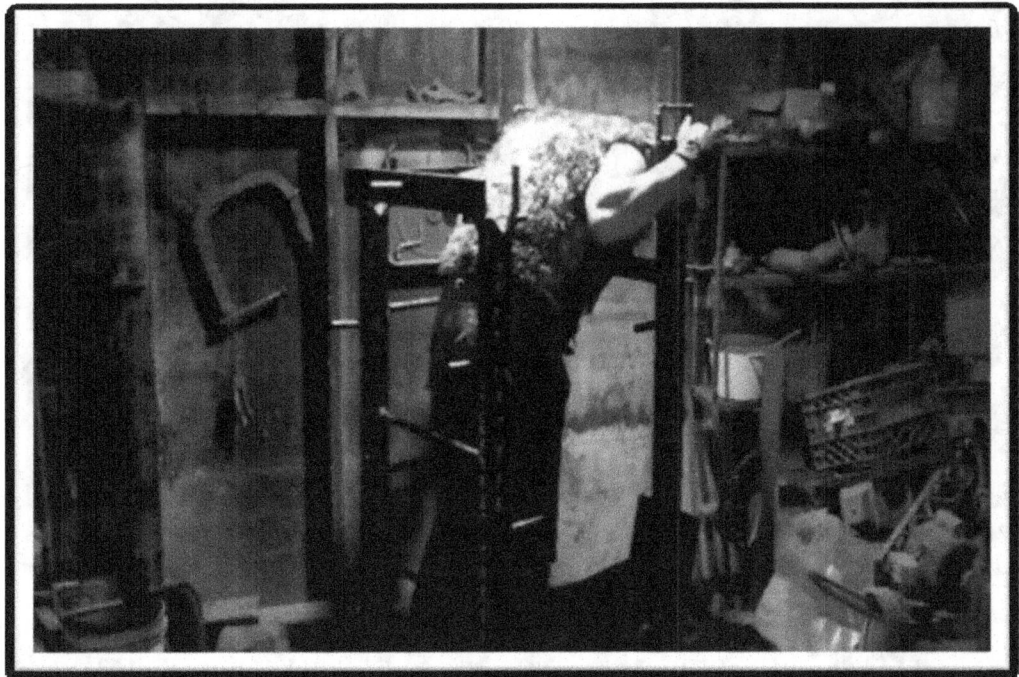

Variation 1: Place your shoulders under the top bar, like if you were to pick a bar off the rack for squats and push the bar up. For me this is set where I would move the bar one to five inches depending on which rack I use. This is one of my favorites for whole body power. You see in the picture here, in the rack, I'm leaning slightly forward, but in my other racks I do the same motion straight up and down or leaning slightly backward.
Variation 2: Do the same quarter squat except this time actively press the bar up as if you were going to push it over your head with your hands. You can use a close or wide grip.

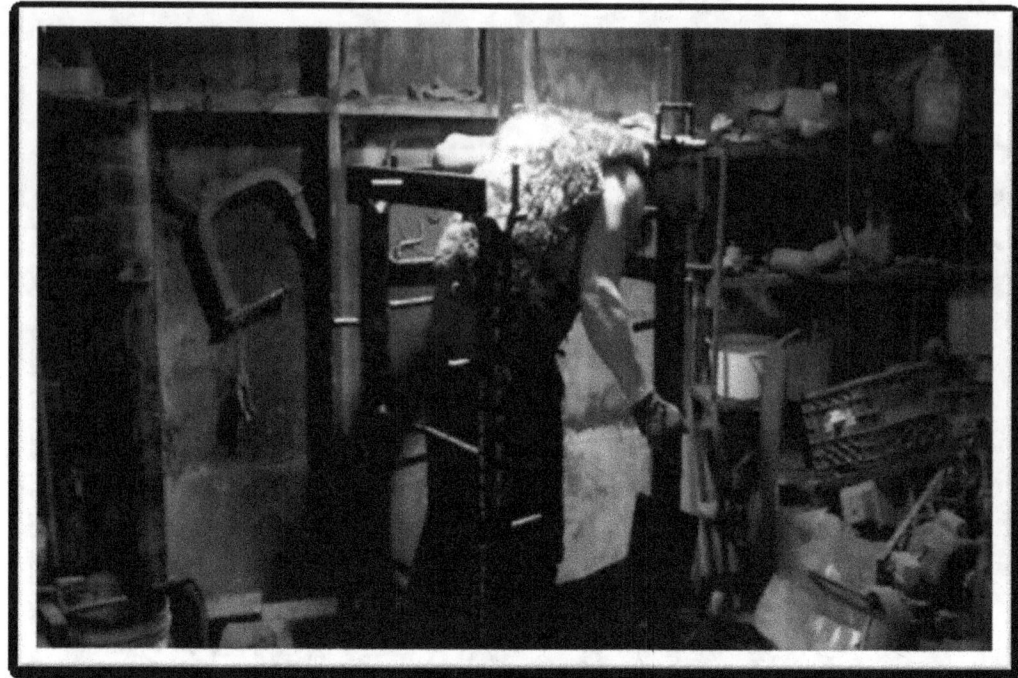

Variation 3: Get back in the original position and twist your hands while you are pushing up.

Variation 4: Twist your legs in while putting the pressure up and out.

Variation 5: Get on your toes, bring one leg forward. Press up and twist in and out.
Variation 6: Push up with the body, but pull down with the hands on the bar.
Variation 7: Push up with the body and one hand on the bar, take the other hand off the bar. You can leave that hand free or push down on another handle or out to the side.
Variation 8: Push up with the body, take both hands off the bar, you can then push out to the side, pull different directions, pull up or down on a different handle with your hands.

Low Squat and Pull

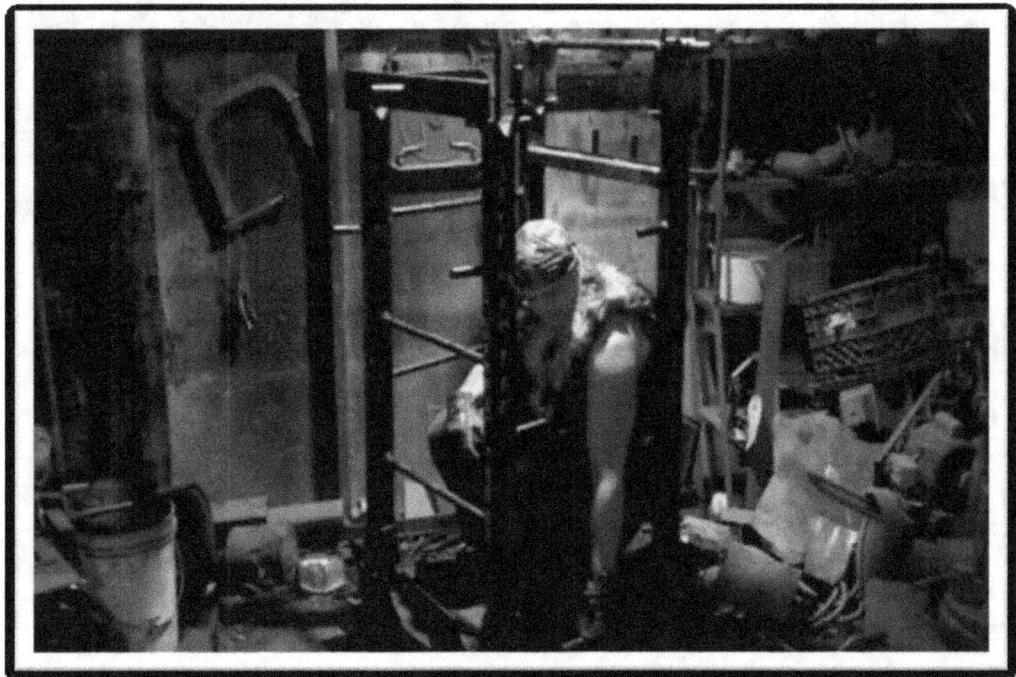

Variation 1: Get yourself into a squat position, this could be low or half squat, knees forward or straight up and down, close or wide, flat footed or on toes. From there grab the a bar or handle with one or two hands, inside or outside the body, close or wide and pull straight up.

Variation 2: Any of the same possible variations, but add pulling in or out pressure with the arms or legs.

Variation 3: Any of the same possible variation, but add pushing forward or pulling back with the arms or legs.

Variation 4: Do any of the squat pull motions but add twisting your wrist in one way or the other while you are doing forward, back, in and out, up or even push down. You can do down & out, down & forward, down & in, down & back – while twisting your wrist all the time.

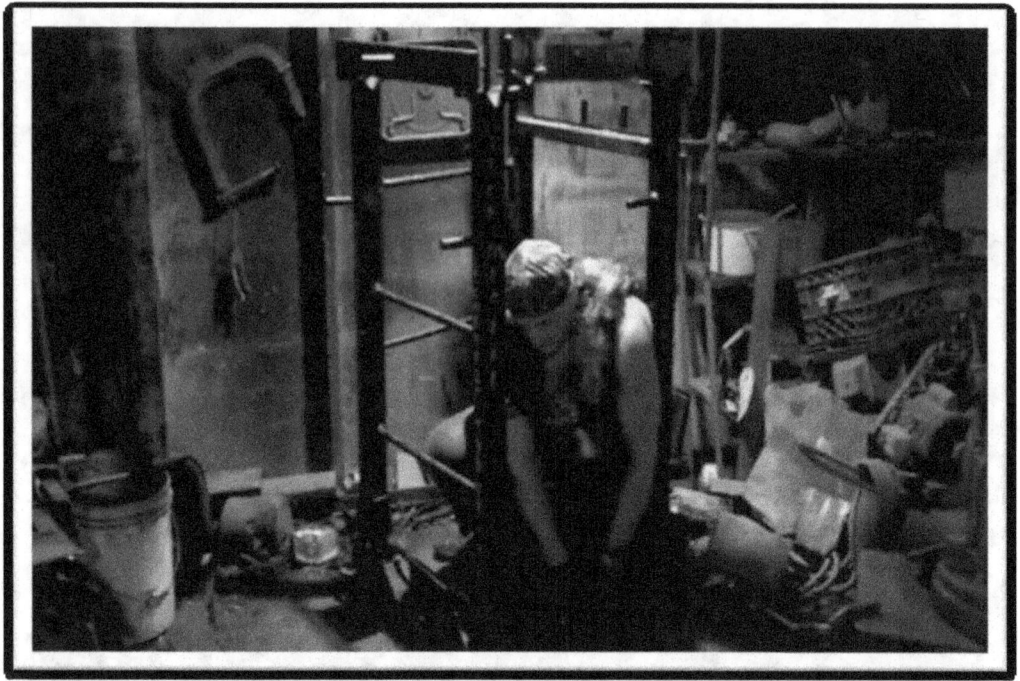

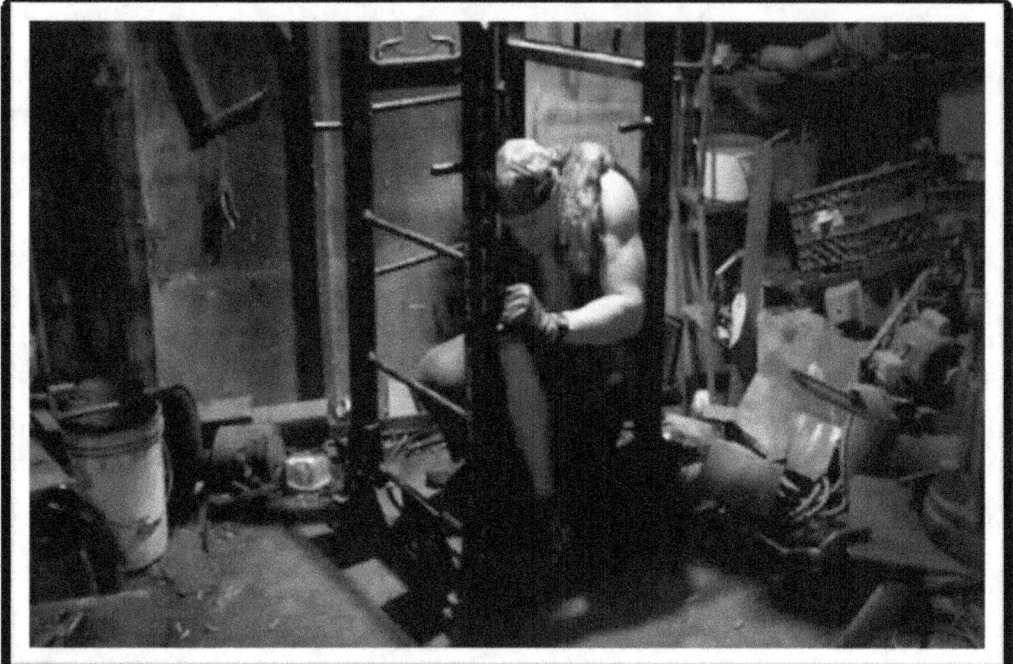

Another Variation: Put your left hand on the middle handle and your right hand on the bottom bar. Pull up with your right hand, as if you want it to meet with your left hand.

Pull Up and Cross your Chest

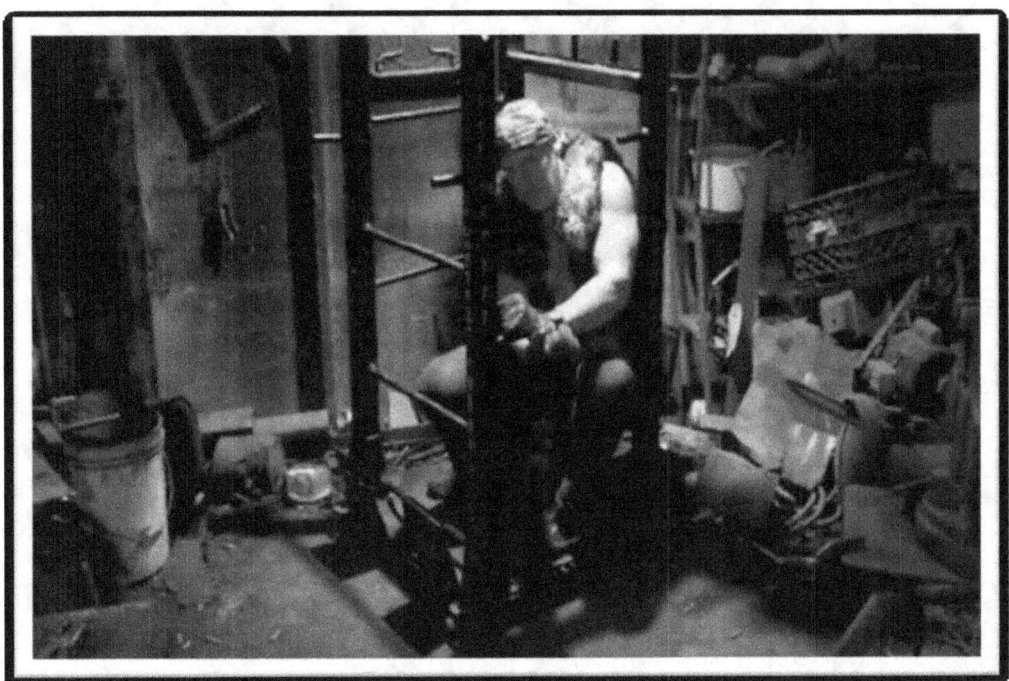

Variation 1: While seated, grab a handle or bar low and to the outside, across your body. Pull straight back as if you're trying to row or pull it across your chest.

Variation 2: Pull up and back or pull up and push forward.

Variation 3: Push down and out, away from your body. Other variations include going down and back, down and forward and down and back while twisting your wrist.

Breaking a bar

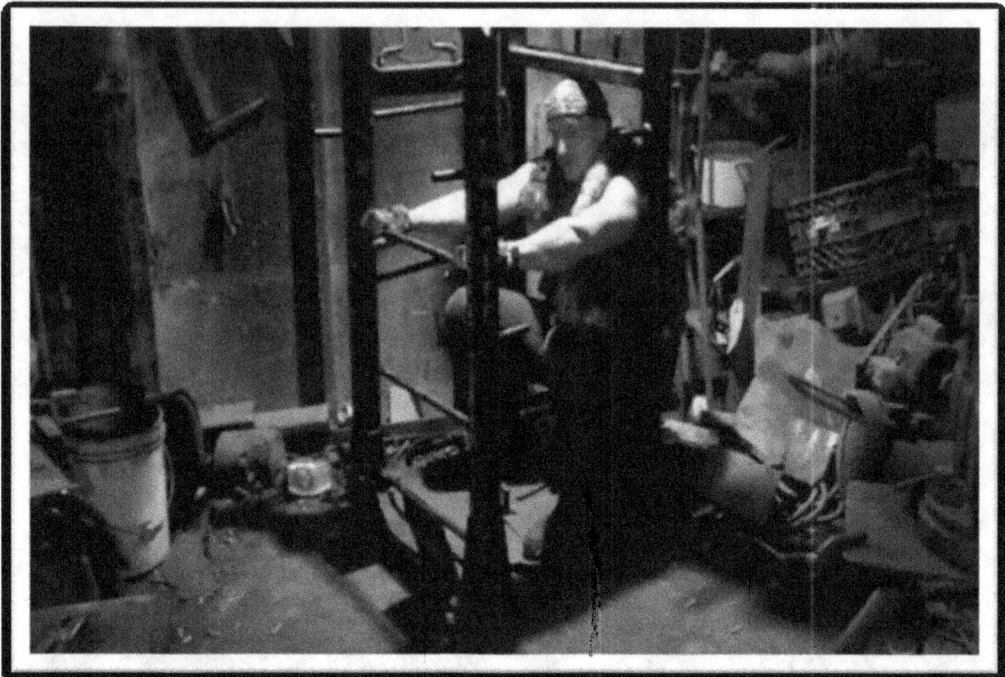

Variation 1: Grab a bar with both hands in a squat or seated position and twist the bar like you want to break it apart.

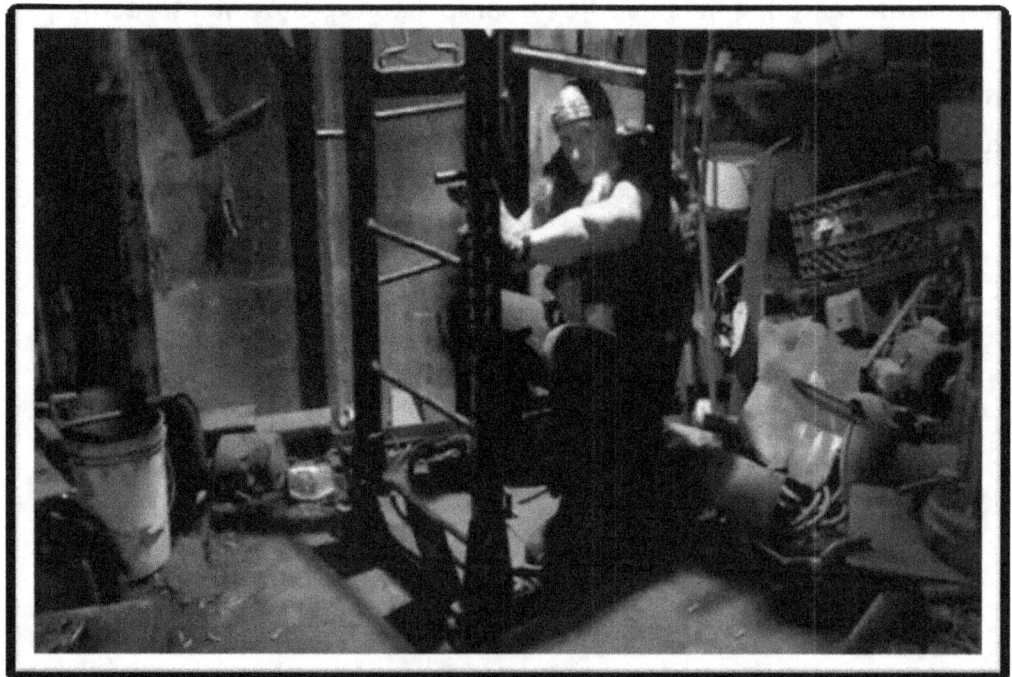

Variation 2: Pull one arm back and push with the other one forward.

Variation 3: Go back and forth, like you are doing jerk reps. Keep going for like 100 jerks or until you get burned. While you are doing back and forth jerks, push your arms in together or push them out. This one is particularly beneficial for your elbow, knees, wrists, ankle and shoulder joints.

Variation 4: Do the same breaking or twisting motion, but vary the height of the bar from lower or higher than the chest and/or lean your bodyweight into the bar or away from the bar as you do the breaking/twisting motion.

Jerks or Isometrics on Toes

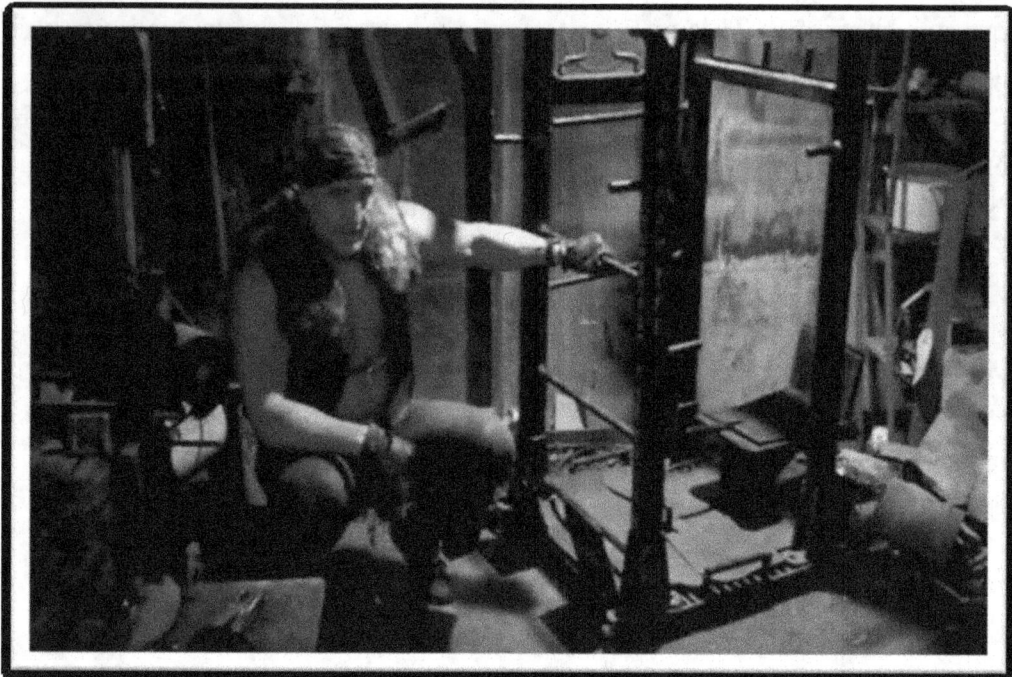

Variation 1: Get down on your toes, grab the bar with one hand and jerk it back and forth. A perfect workout for ankles, feet and knees. Alternately you can hold for time or any of the isometric styles you prefer.

Variation 2: Grab the bar with both hands (see Variation 1 image) and go back and forth, while you are still on your toes.

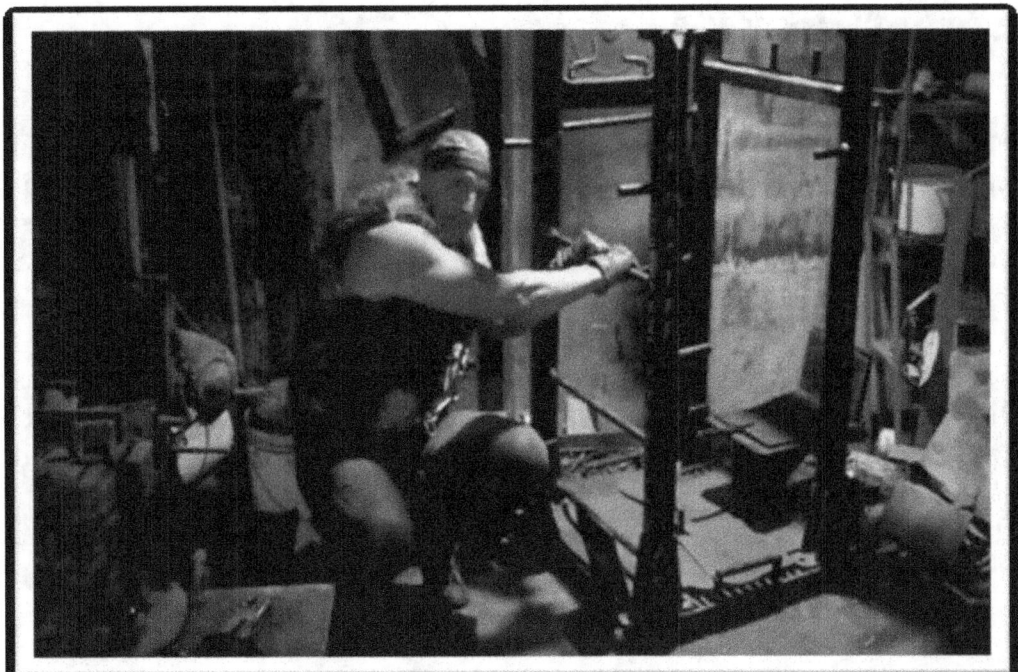

Variation 3: While in the same position, pull up or push down, jerk the bar to the sides or try to push both arms forward and/or back.

Variation 4: Vary the width of your feet or the grip on the bar, also vary by standing on the toes on one foot at a time, which the other is flat or just on one foot if you can.

Exercises with a Classic Isometric Rack

This section will contain some of my favorite exercises and the wild stuff you can do with what we call a Classic Isometric rack. Many of the old time racks such as the York Barbell racks and the earlier isometric devices were very simple and built along the lines of the rack I have built here. You will see it has three major bars that slide in and out at varying heights across two pieces of telephone pole which I sunk in the ground.

This particular rack also has a couple of low round rings mounted to it to do work very close to the ground. It also has a specialty gripper that I use for isometrics, which is two bars welded across a section of car spring that allows me to do compressions and squeezes similar to a very heavy gripper. This rack is very convenient and easy to do many of the exercises we've already shown such as the quarter squats and deadlifts, but it was an almost unlimited variety of exercises you can do on it.

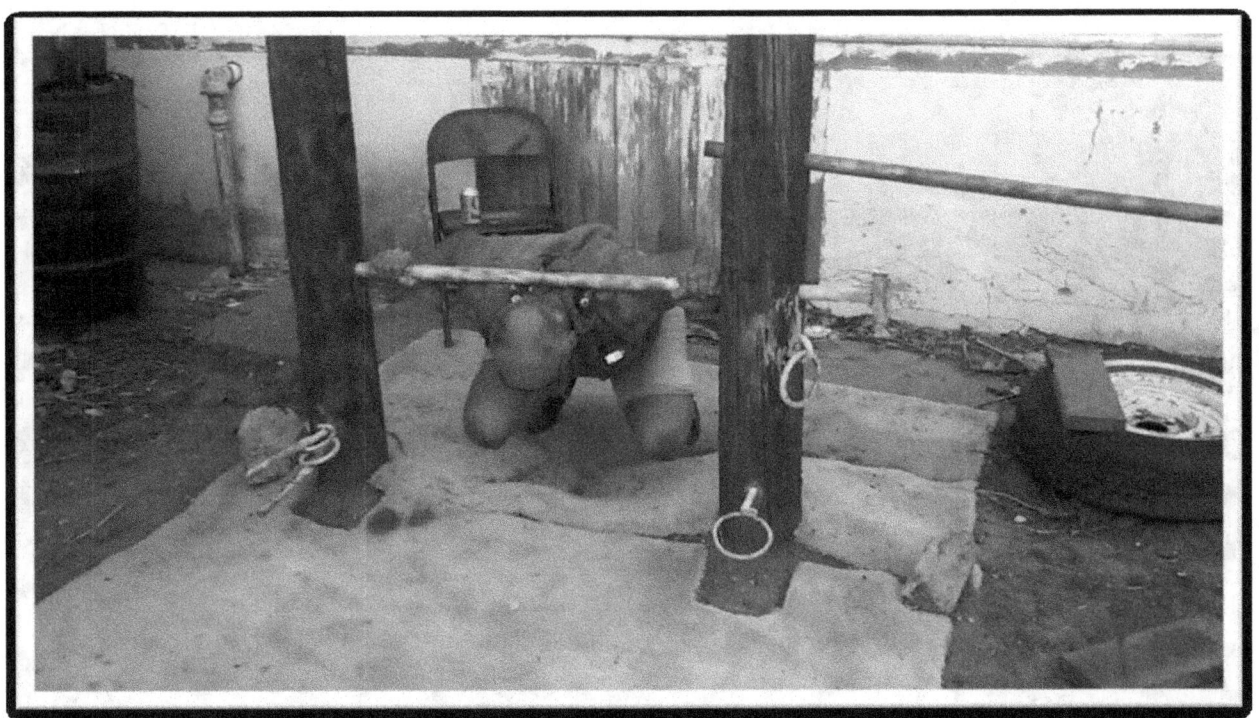

Super Low Squat

Variation 1: Set the bar as low as you can possibly squeeze under in a squat position. Get under, put the bar against your shoulders and push up.

Variation 2: Perform the low squat by pushing forward and up.

Variation 3: Perform the low squat while on toes

Variation 4: Perform the low squat and twist the bar with the hands – up, back down and forward.

Variation 5: Perform the low squat and twist the body to the side or attempt to push the rack straight side ways while in the low squat.

Variation 6: Vary the width and angles your feet and twist the feet and knees in and out as you push.

Hands in Front - Push and Pull Against the Bar with Various Stances and Body Positions

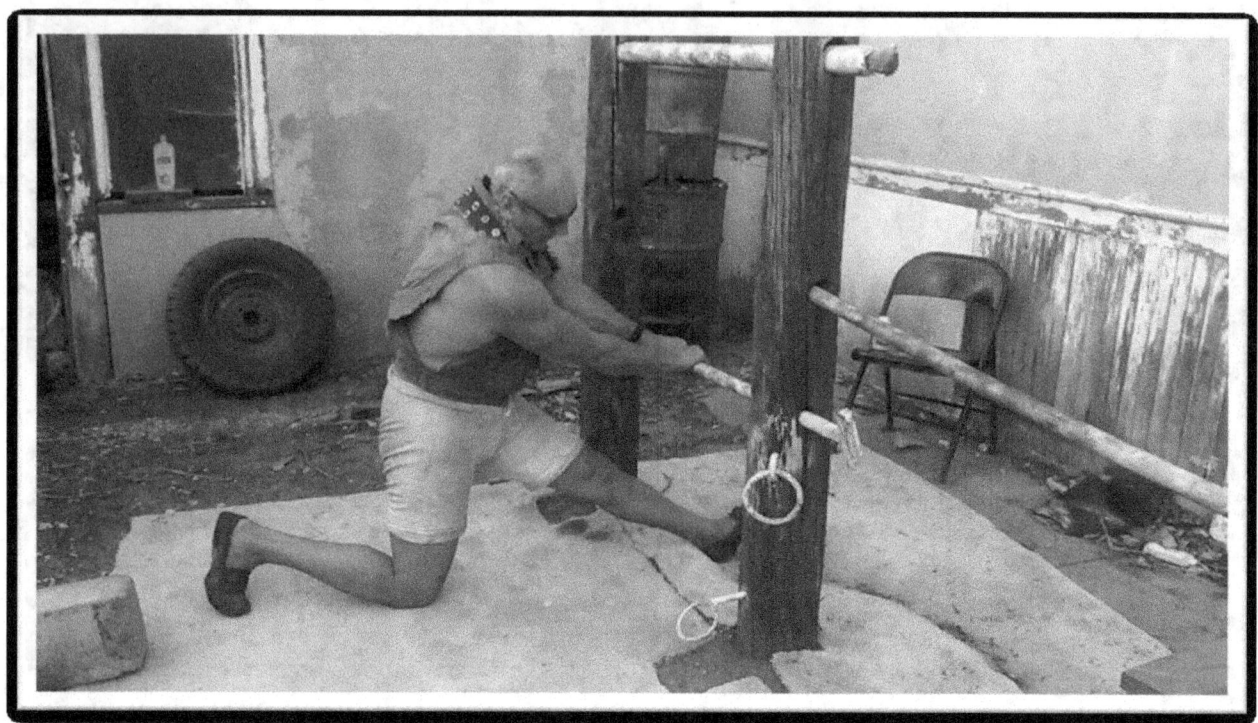

Half Kneeling Push and Pull

All of the following variations apply to the next several forward pushing and pulling exercises shown in the pictures. The only difference is the basic stance or body angle that you use. This includes the half kneeling stance above, the stretched out stance in the following photo and the standing stance in the picture after. However all of the hand positions and forward/backward, up and down, multiple directions apply to every one of the stances.

Variation 1: Assume the half kneeling or down on one knee position. You can use the classic position or the one shown in the picture with one leg stretched out straight forward bracing. Grab one of the bars and push or pull forward or backward.
Variation 2: Push forward with one hand, pull back with the other at the same time.
Variation 3: Push forward and up or down or side to side at the same time.
Variation 4: Pull backward and up or down or side to side at the same time.
Variation 5: Push forward or pull backward while one hand pulls up and the other pushes down.
Variation 6: Vary the width of your hands from wide all the way to close and even crossing each other to hit different muscles.

Variation 7: Instead of pushing with the hands straight forward from the body, but the hands are grabbing the bar out to the side and push forward or pull back and up, down or to the side.

45 Degrees Stretched Out or Plank Style Push and Pull

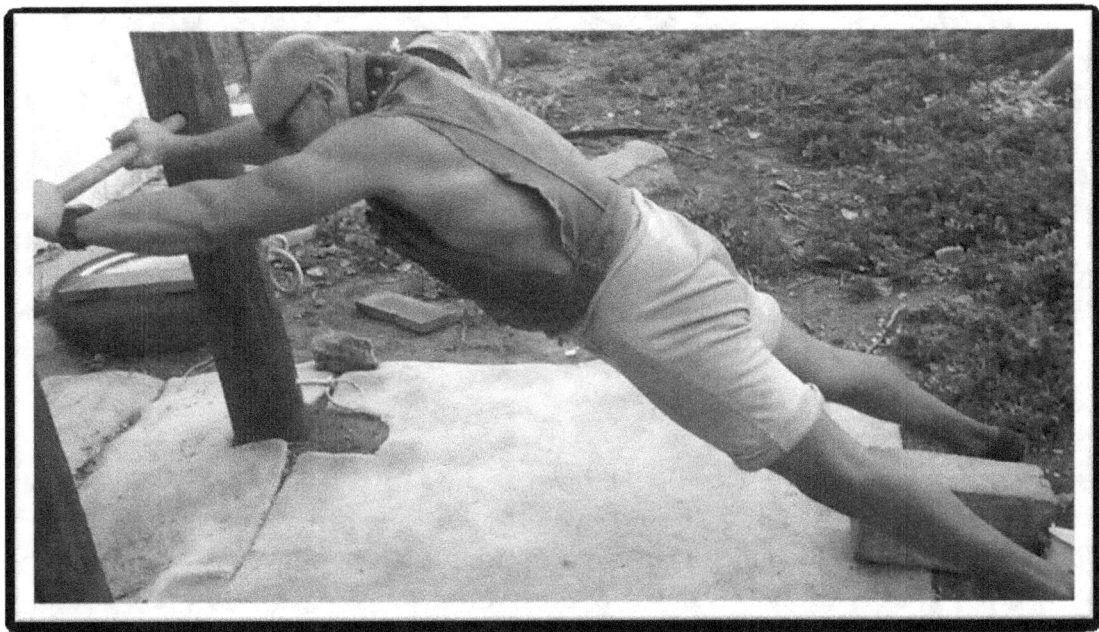

Standing Split Stance Push or Pull *(Can also be done with a basic feet directly under shoulders, feet even, stance.)*

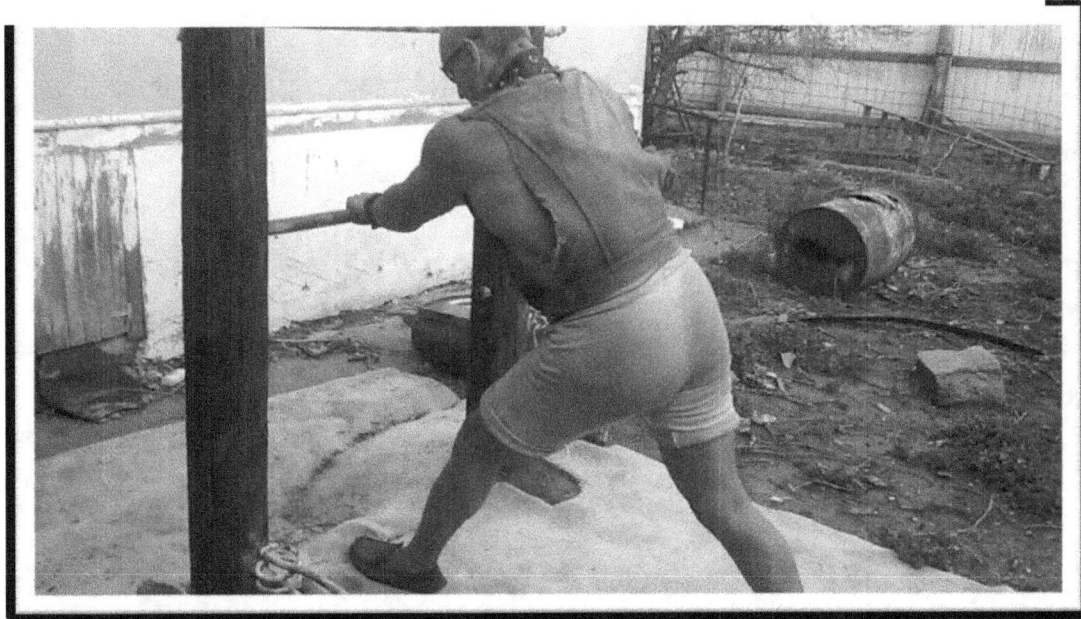

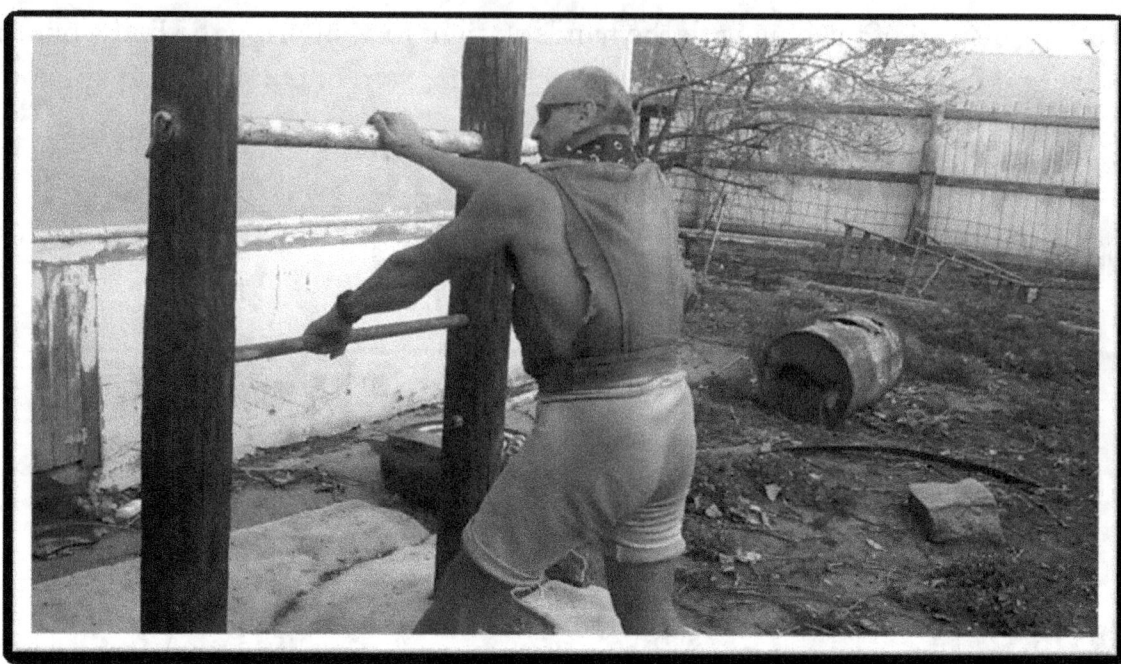

Two Bar or Two Angle Push and Pulls

There are too many variations here to list. However these two pictures show just two of the possibilities. The first one I'm grabbing two different height bars, the second I'm grabbing the high bar with my hand wrapped around it and pushing or pulling into the post with my other hand. All these carry the same variations as the front push and pulls. That is – they can be done from multiple stances, kneeling, half kneeling, split stance, etc., and all the other pressure variations apply as well. Push, pull, twist, up, down, forward, backward and wrist twisting for an unlimited number of variations.

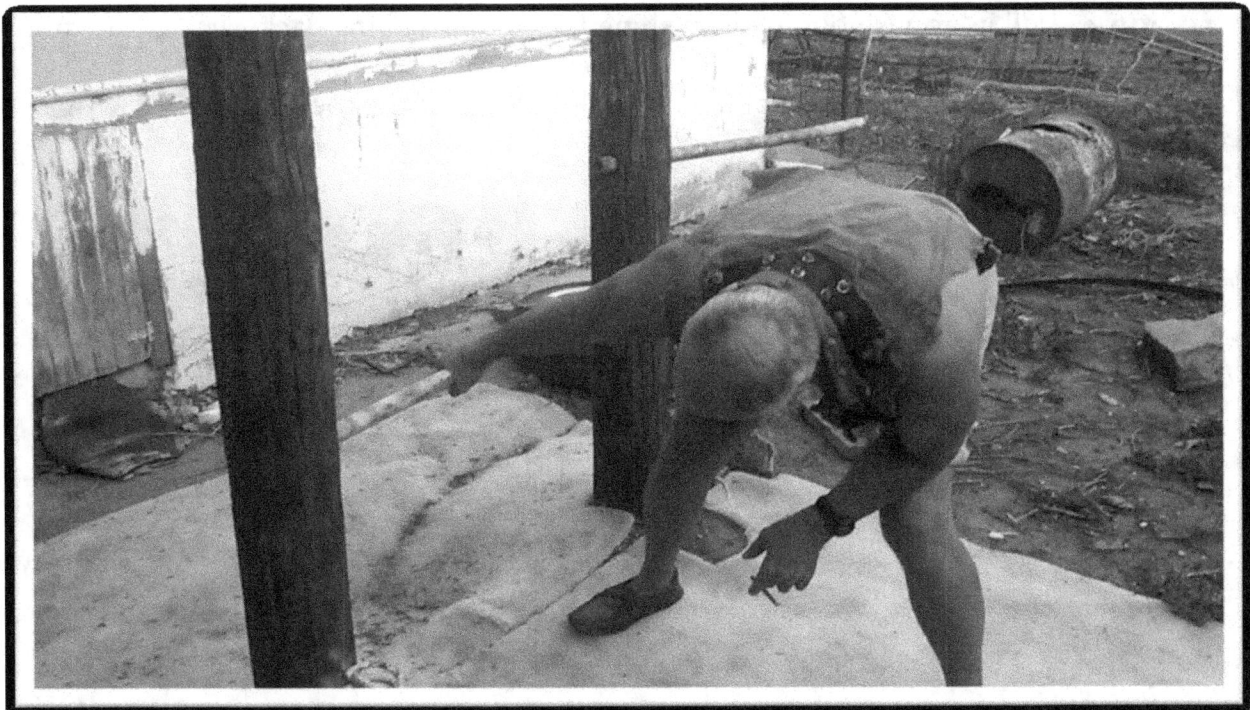

Bent Forward Outside the Body Push and Pull

Variation 1: This is excellent for training the side waist as well as chest and back. Grab a low bar as far out to the side as you can reach in fully bent position. Pull into the body or push away.

Variation 2: Pull in and up or down at the same time

Variation 3: Push out and up or down at the same time.

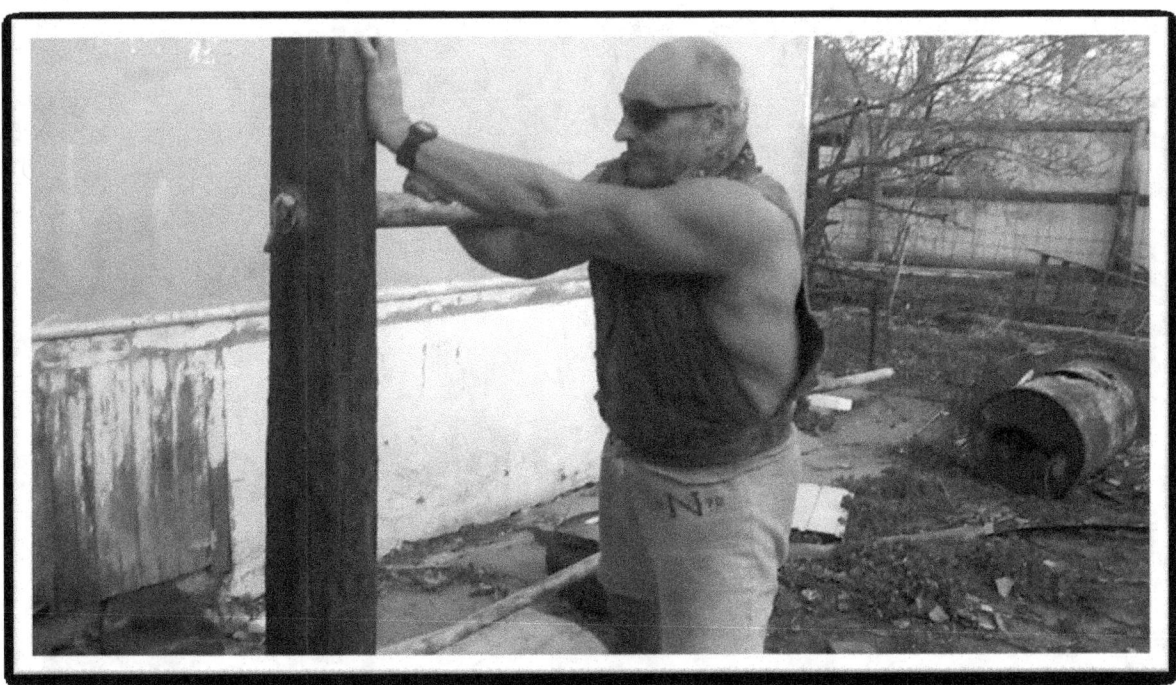

Variation 4: Pull in or push out while pushing forward or pulling backward at the same time

Variation 5: Do the bent forward pull while holding the on the toes position or with a narrow or wide stance.

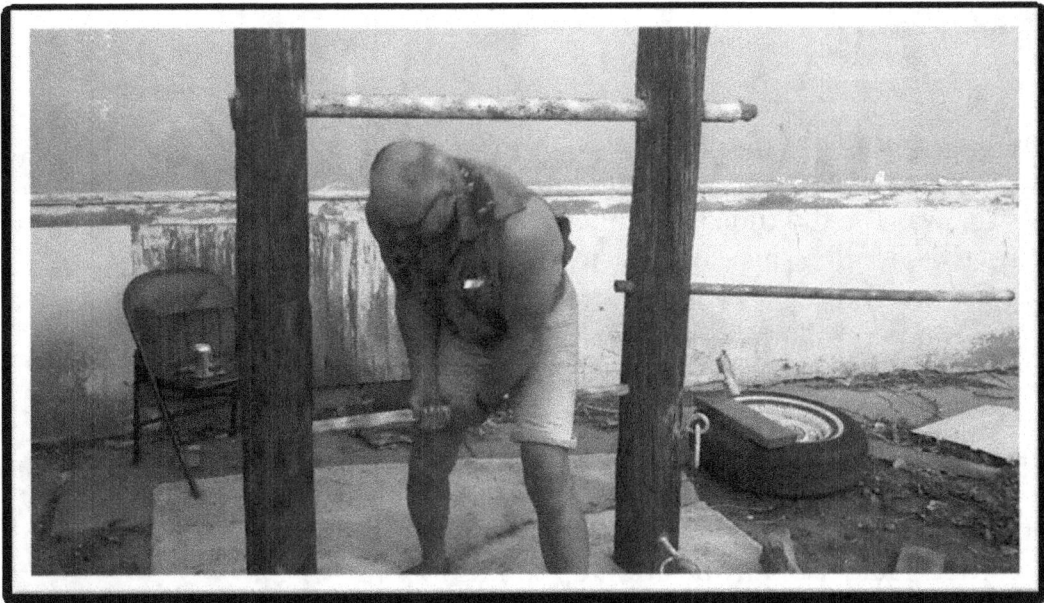

Jefferson Style Pulls

Again there are almost limitless variations here. These are named after the Jefferson lift which is done by straddling a barbell and lifting it. Similar to the position I am in over the bottom bar of the isometric rack. In the pictures you see a narrow stance, hands in front and a wide stance back against the post variation. You can also do the classic Jefferson variation where one hand is in front of the body and the other is behind and as with all the other isometrics we've taught so far there is the multiple variation directions of pull up, push down, pull with one hand, push with the other, pull up and twist left or right, pull up and push forward or back, close grip, wide grip, and on the toes positions.

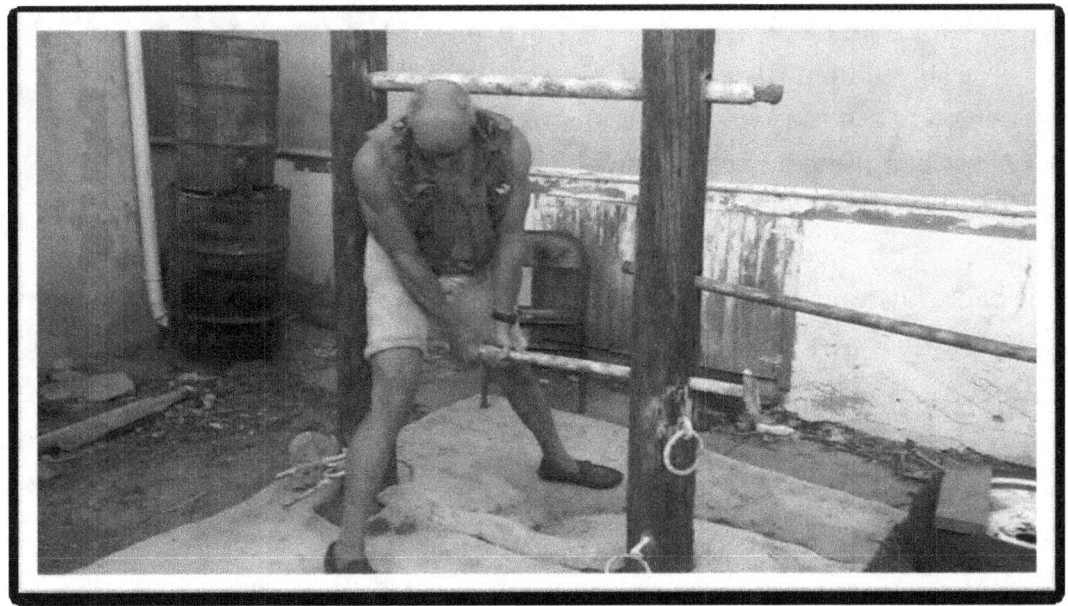

Pressing Isometric

This is one of my favorite pressing isometrics because it's a one armed variation similar to how you would support a weight in one hand like in a bent press the way the old time strongmen did. Really tones the shoulder muscles and side muscles of the body. Teaches you how to graft the elbow to hip and put the hip out to the side for pressing power. We've shown pressing and pulling to the front, but overhead is just as important and all the variations apply. One arm, two arm, to the side, front or curl grip, in front or behind the neck, kneeling, standing, squatting, starting off the shoulder or any position up to full lock out. Also add in the twists and multiple direction work of pressing up, but going forward or backward, twisting left or right or any combination of those simultaneously.

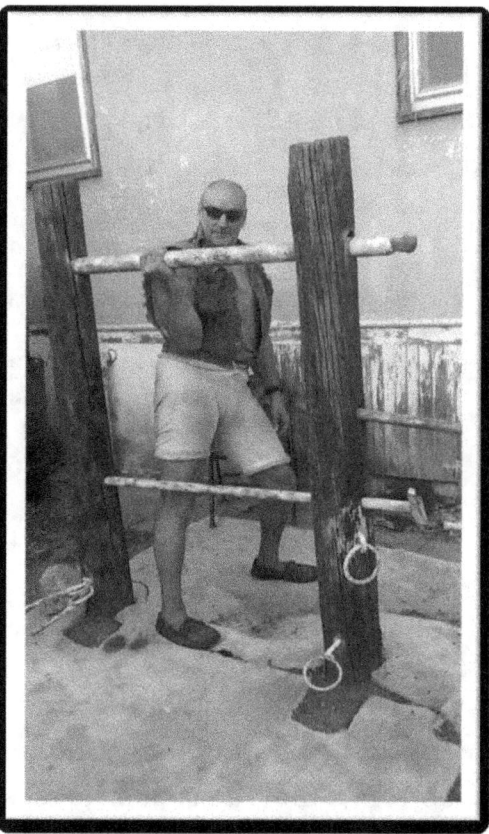

One Shoulder Quarter Squat with Press Variation

This is an example of a quarter squat, but done with the bar on one shoulder, body turned to the side. In this particular one you can see I'm using a pressing variation with my hands and neck, both pushing up with my body as well as driving up with my arms and hands, at a 45 degree angle away from my body while simultaneously pushing up with the neck. This hits a ton of muscles. It also opens the other variations of pulling down with the hands instead of pushing up while keeping pressure pushing upward with the body. Also pushing forward or back, pushing left or right. One hand up, one hand down, one leg and multiple foot stances.

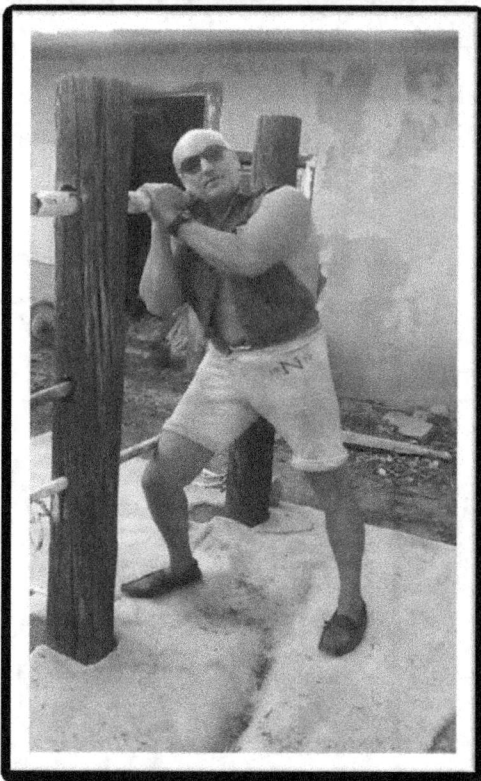

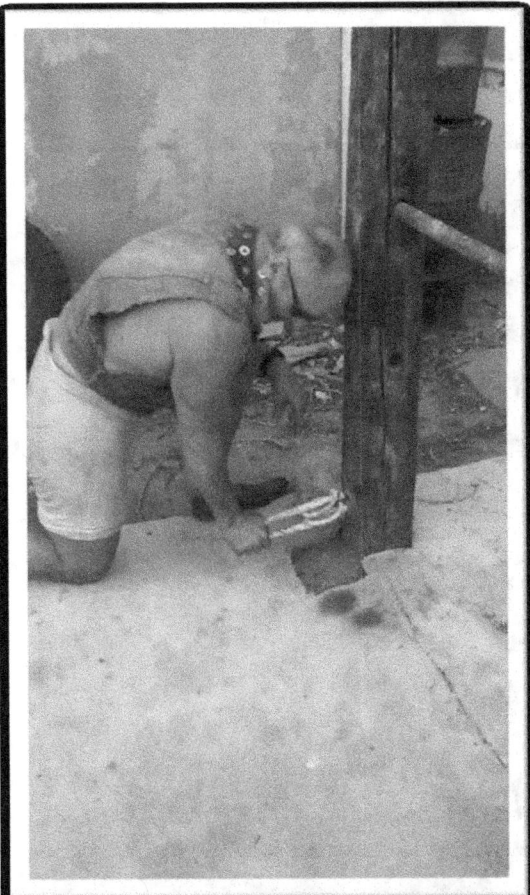

Isometric Gripper

Much of the grip in your hands is actually isometric power. The ability to hold on to barbells, rugged surfaces, the ability to squeeze them and keep hold is an isometric for your hand. I purposely built this gripper piece with long handles so I could simply adjust the tension by grabbing it shorter or longer. I also do various holds for length of time and often use my body to crush the ends together and then hold until my fingers give out. I often also work on different positions of the hand or arm and flex different arm muscles while squeezing it.

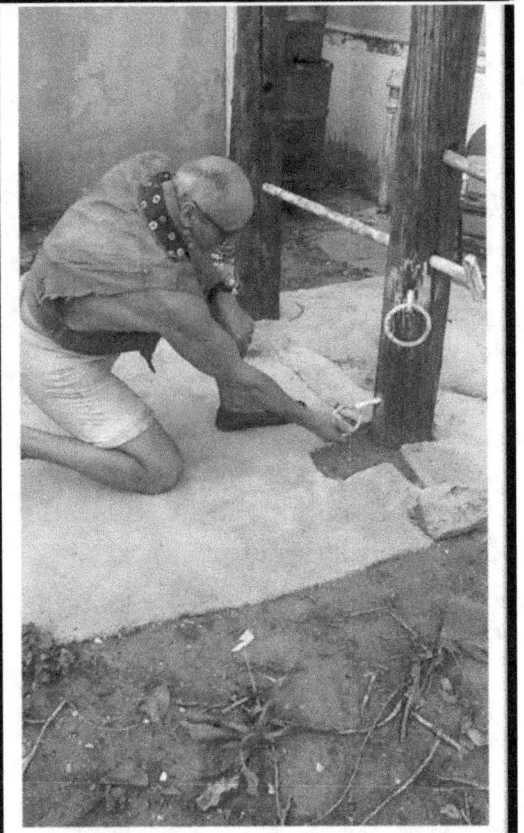

Ultra Low Position Pulls

This ring is useful for pulling in very low positions, developing flexibility and pulling in longer than normal ranges. You never know when you may need to be strong standing up or stretched all the way out till your fingers are on the ground. I like to use this one for pulling back like a one arm row, but also by adding different twists such as pulling up and back or up and forward or up and to the side or twisting my hand upside down and pulling from there.

Exercises with my Isometric Arm Wrestling Table

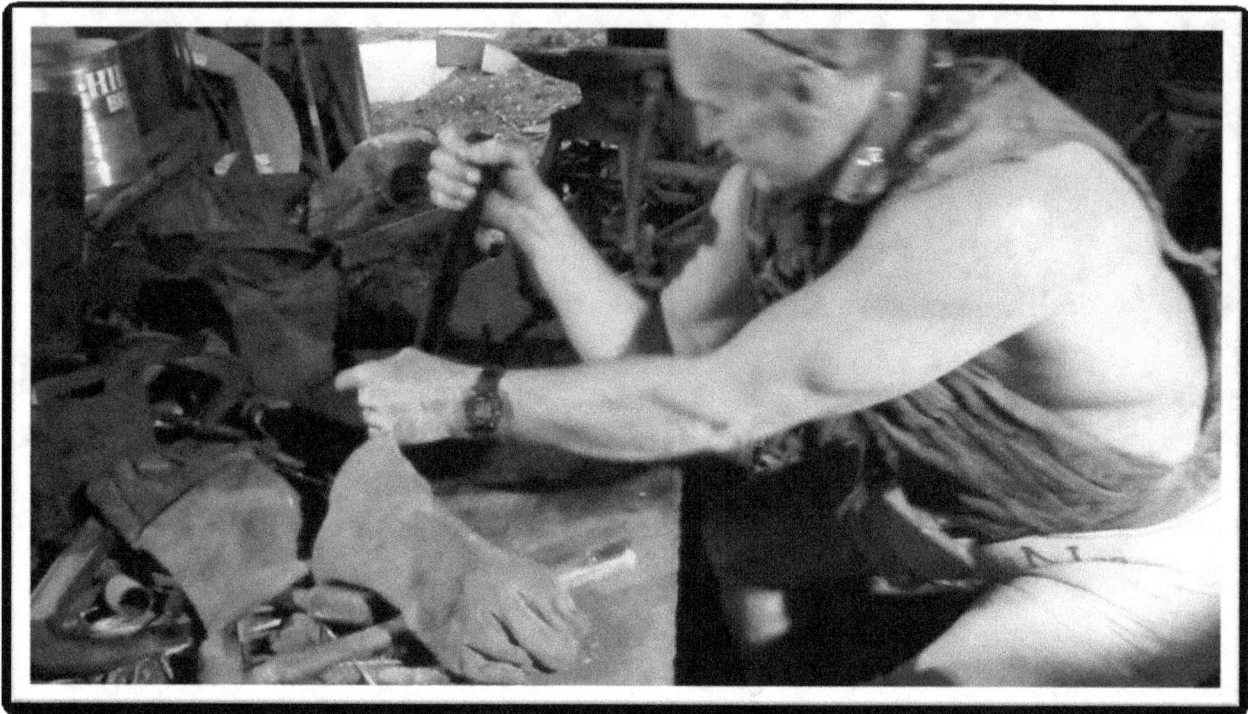

Many people don't know I use to arm wrestle a lot and actually sold a spring arm wrestling device for a while back in the mail order days, before the internet. Arm wrestling in itself is a great workout and develops not just the arms but the whole upper body. So I had this steel work table in my shed and I welded two short pegs and a long bar at the angle of a human arm to the top of the table. It lets me really work my arms as well as stay in shape to arm wrestle if I feel like it. Part of the reason this is so good for arm wrestling and makes you so strong is that arm wrestling is basically a high intensity partner isometric. And it puts your hand, arm and body into hundreds of different positions. Shown here is the basic starting position, off hand on the short peg and wrestling arm on the long post. From there and in all the following arm wrestling pictures I always try to work as many angles and combinations of directions as I can think of. Pushing straight forward, pulling straight back, pushing and pulling to the side, twisting the wrist over and simulating actual arm wrestling techniques or positions. I apply the same methods to these that I do the other isometrics, some max, some jerk reps, some timed holds, switching positions as fast as possible and working back and forth between left and right hand.

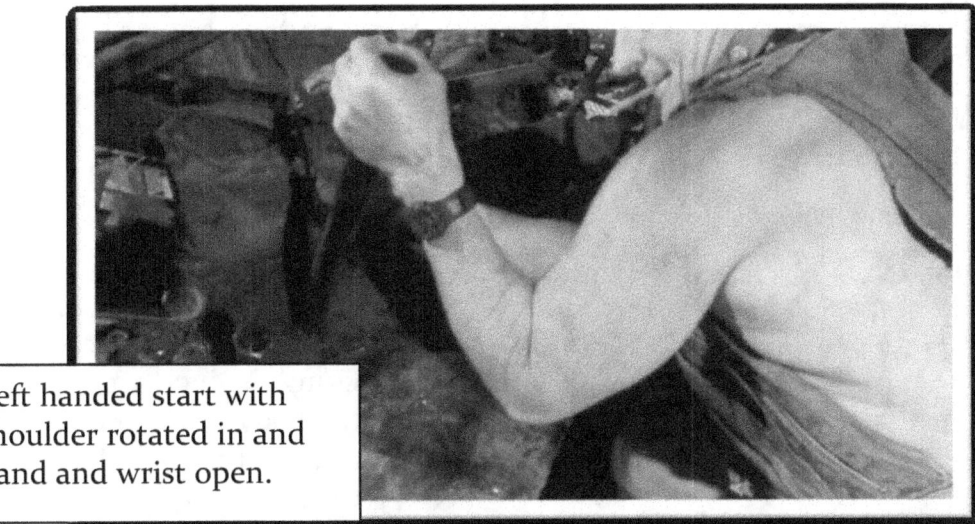

Left handed start with shoulder rotated in and hand and wrist open.

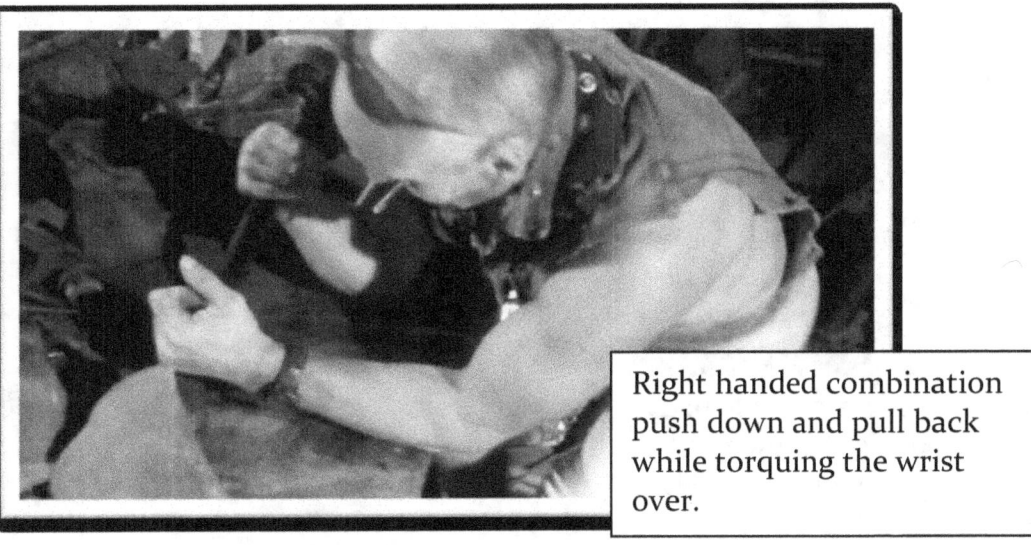

Right handed combination push down and pull back while torquing the wrist over.

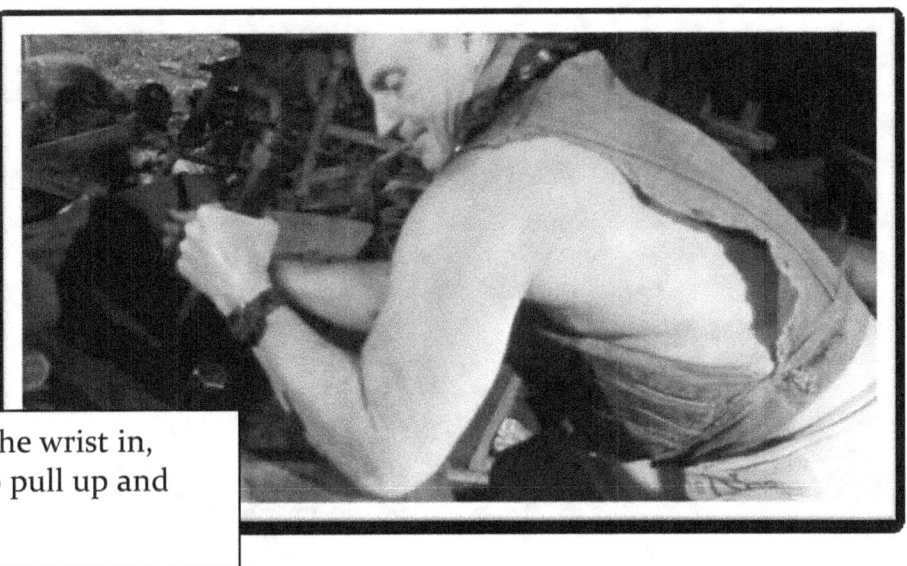

Twisting the wrist in, starting to pull up and back.

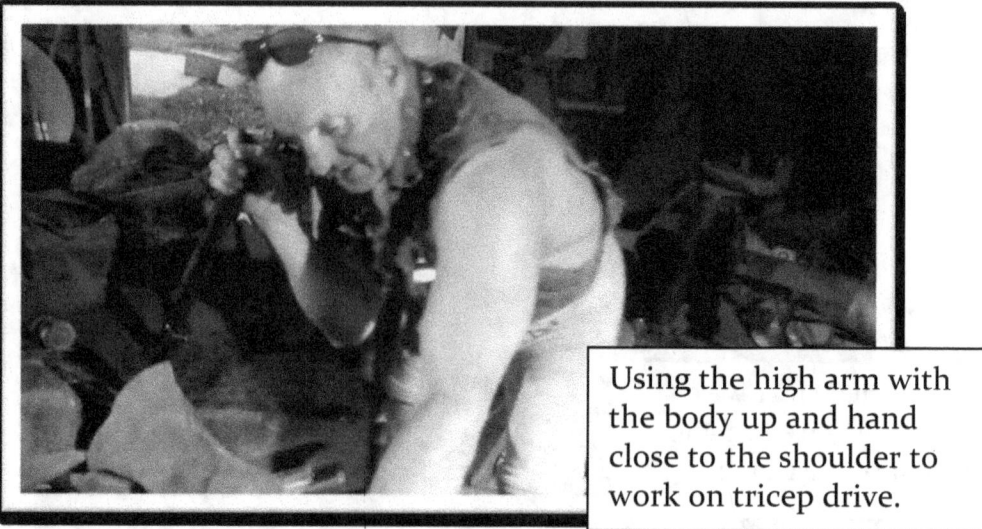

Using the high arm with the body up and hand close to the shoulder to work on tricep drive.

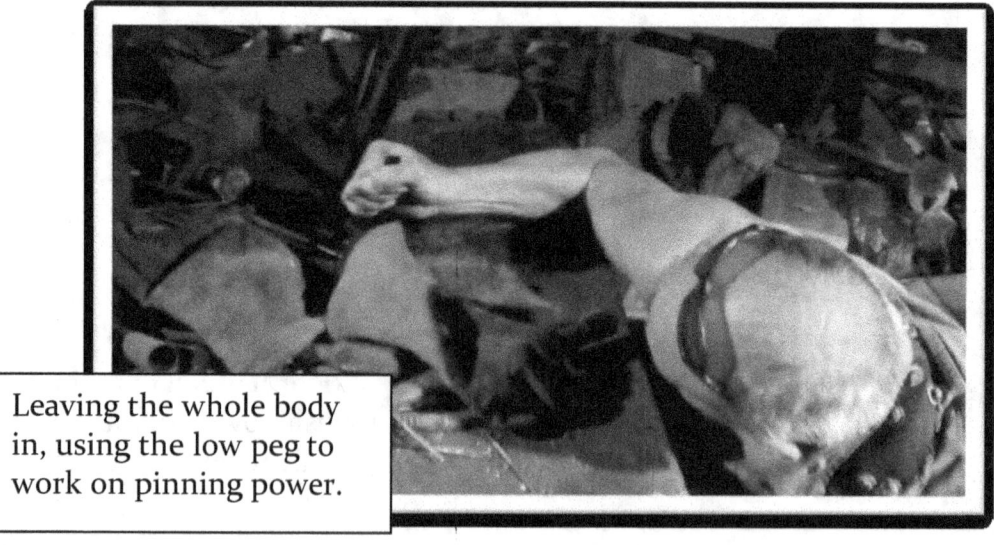

Leaving the whole body in, using the low peg to work on pinning power.

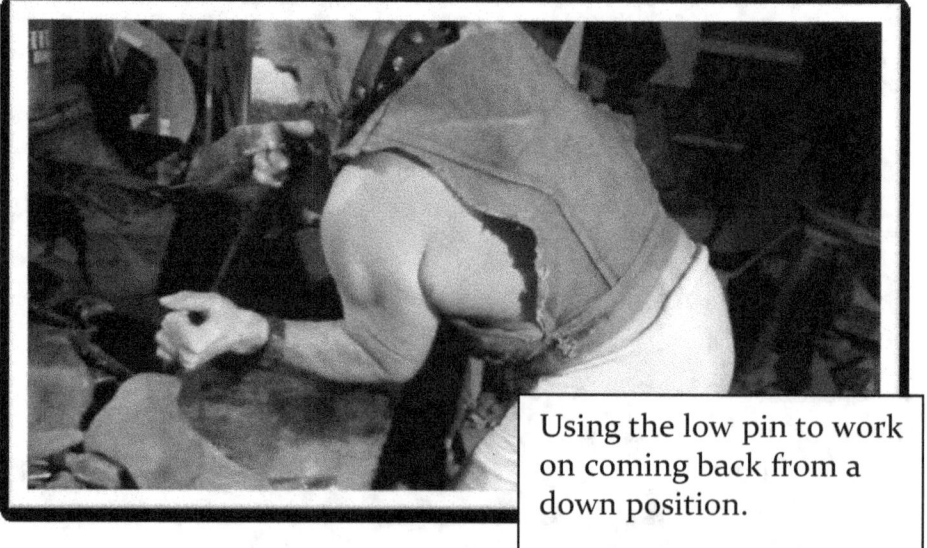

Using the low pin to work on coming back from a down position.

Isometrics on Every Day Objects

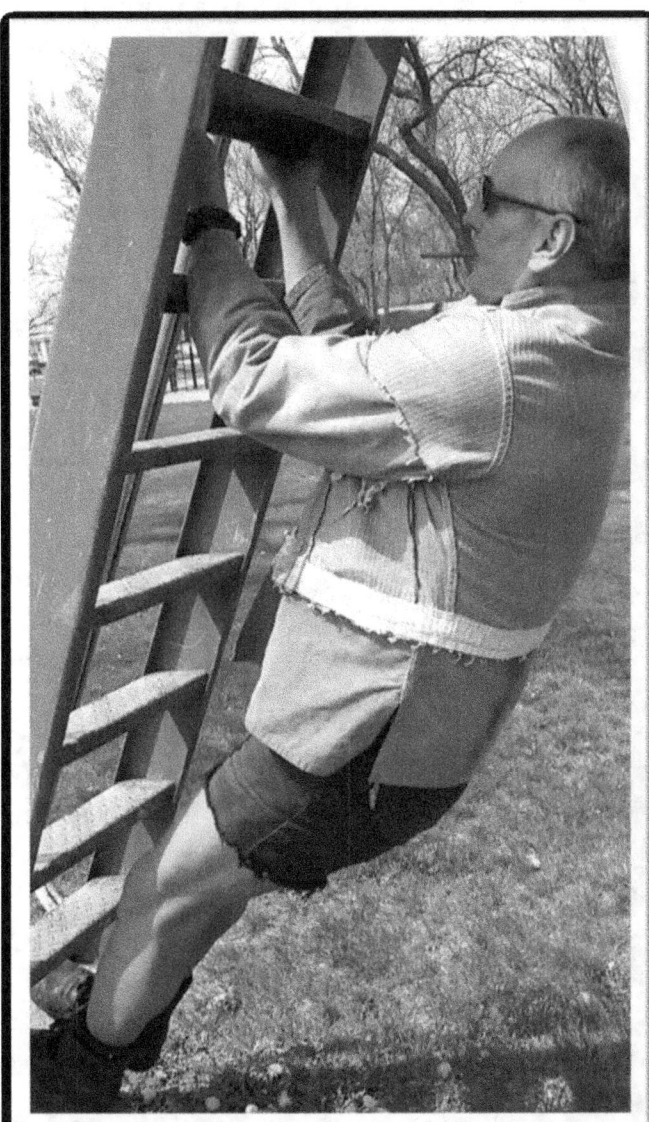

One of the great things about isometrics is that you can use just about anything to do them on. Especially if you're paying attention to your surroundings and you're creative. I like to get outside and go to the park and use different equipment to do isometrics there. As well as anything stationary. Telephone poles, heavy equipment, farm equipment, trees, stadium steps, the possibilities and the workouts are endless. In the picture here I'm doing isometrics on a ladder from a playground slide.

This is a little different from the normal isometric I do, because I'm actually supporting my bodyweight, but I'm also pulling against the ladder steps. Again – pushing and pulling, forward and back, up and down and twisting side to side. The square grips of the steps also give you some unique opportunities to work your fingers in unusual positions.

Simulated Back Lift Isometric

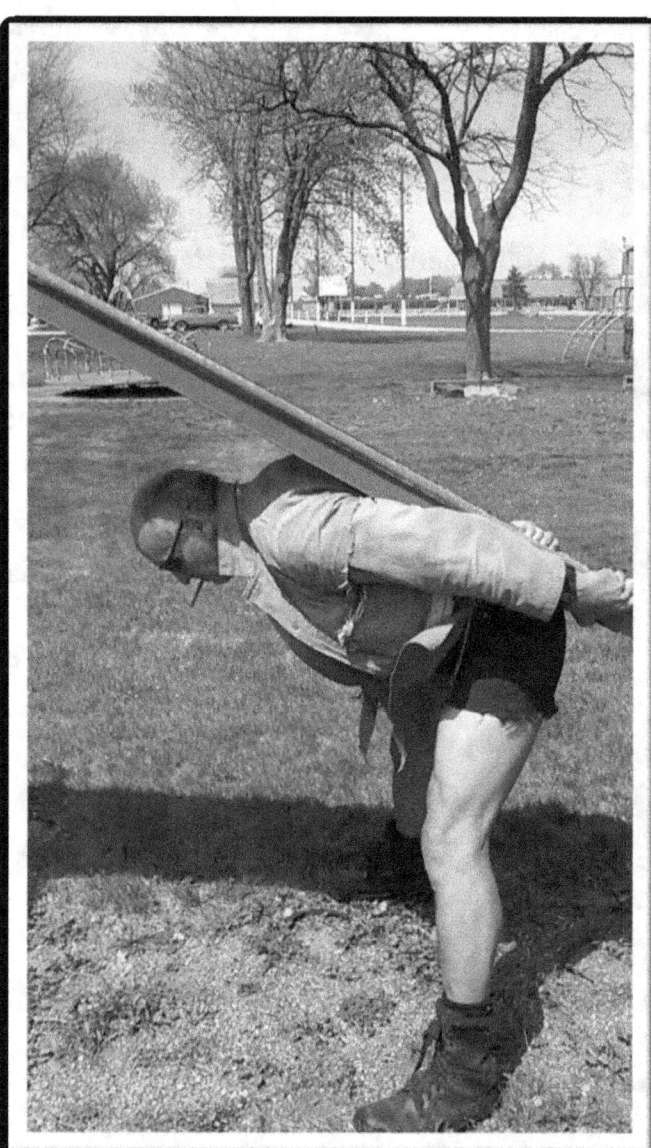

This is one of my favorite isometrics, because it's close to one of my favorite actual lifts – the back lift. I even have a set of bars welded on my specialty isometric rack to practice this same position. You can develop an immense amount of strength with this exercise while developing all the joints of the lower body, and the hips, legs and back. I'm using a slide here, because an anchored slide provides a great, easy way to practice this. Be careful though – if it isn't anchored, you'll pull it out of the ground. I practiced this with close and wide stance and twisting my feet and legs in and out, or driving one leg forward and back.

Single Sided Good Morning with Multiple Direction Push

This next piece of playground equipment is great because it has bars welded, vertical and horizontal at low, medium and tall heights as well as an arc. So you can do hundreds of angles. One we haven't shown is this good morning exercise which essentially puts your upper back against a bar and you push up as if trying to stand up with a bar. This variation has the bar on only one shoulder or side of my body so it really torques not on the back and hips, but the side abdominals as well. At the same time I'm also pushing and pulling on the low horizontal and vertical bars to create extra pressure in different directions and I'm also driving my feet and shoulders in different directions while pushing up.

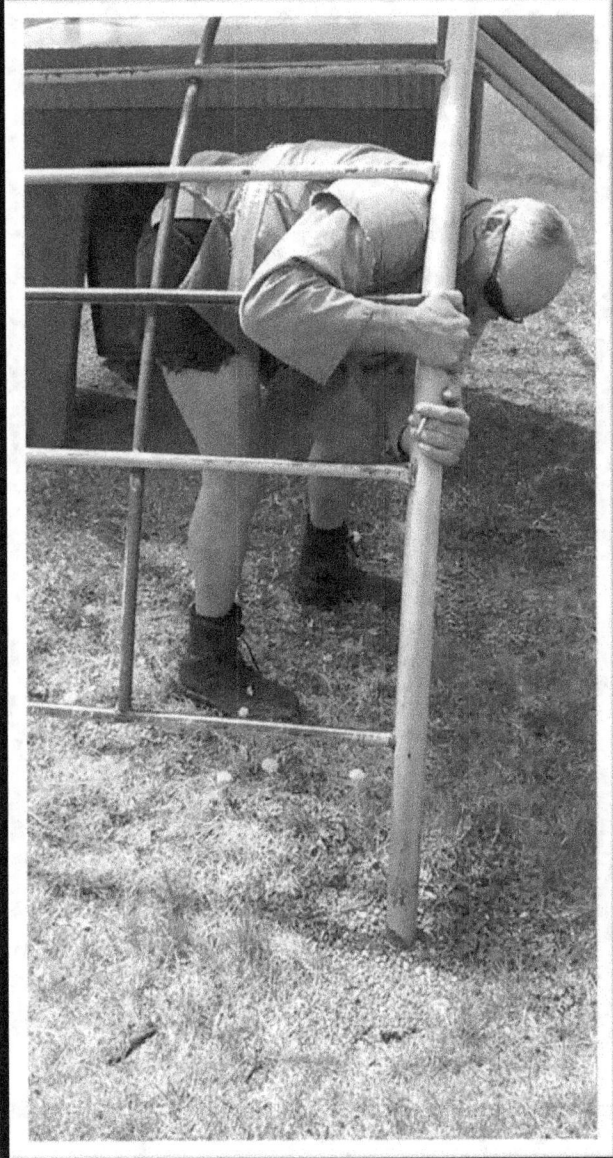

Ultra Wide Stance Vertical and Horizontal Squat Push

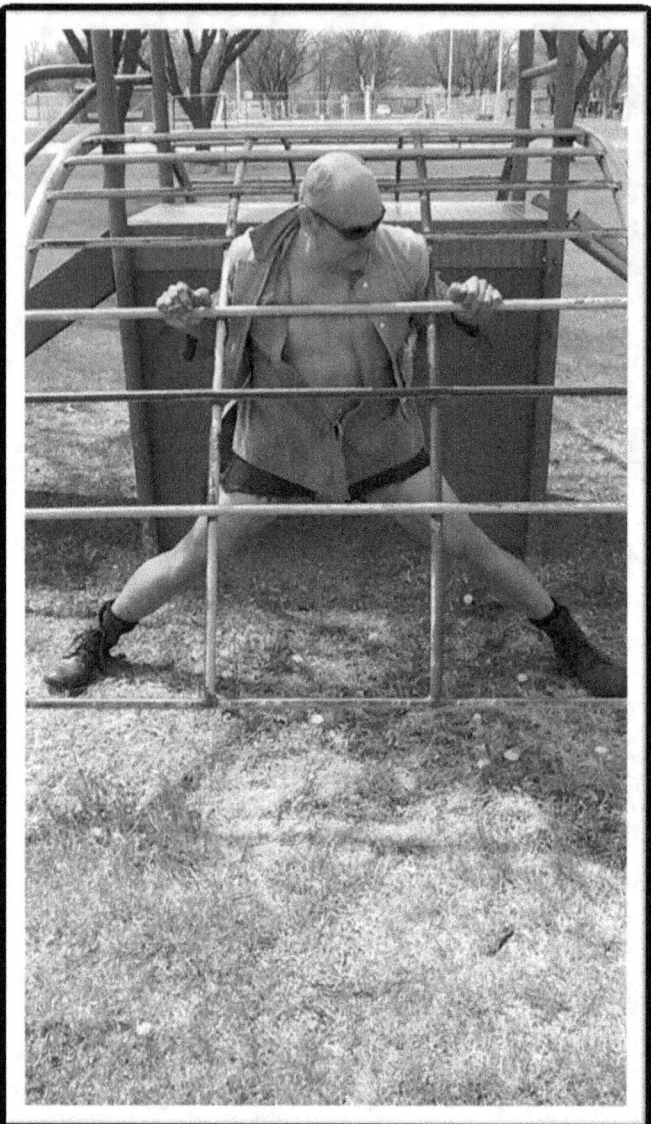

This is a better picture of that particular jungle gym equipment which give you the perfect opportunity to do every angle of squat press or pull or anything else you can think of. This is a very wide stance squat push where I'm doing what's akin to a front squat, but pushing up and out at the same time.

Also if you notice there's a bar directly behind my back so I keep my hands on that bar and switch from dropping to a front squat to dipping my shoulders under the bar for a back squat and pushing up with my body and hands. I also lean my body back into the bar behind me simulating a bench press.

Telephone Pole Isometrics and Bear Hugs

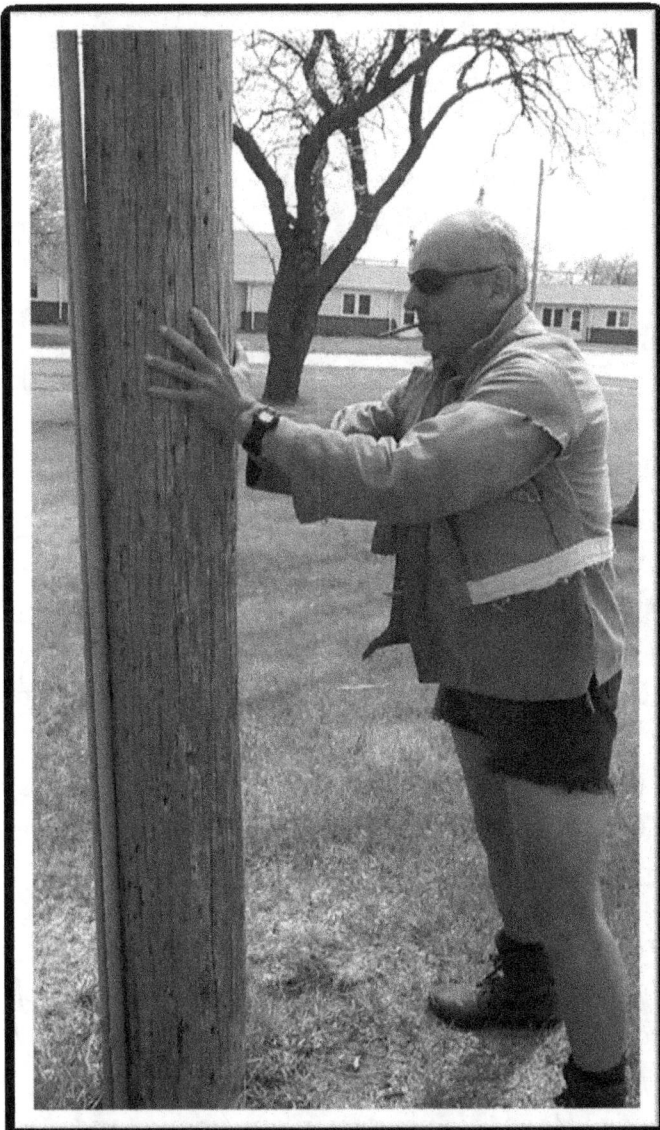

These are one of my favorites because telephone poles are just everywhere! They're great for training the bear hug which is a basic test of human strength. Many of the things lifted in the real world have to be bear hugged to be picked up, and if you've ever wrestled you know the importance of that kind of squeezing strength.

Here I'm just starting to practice by using my hands straight forward to squeeze the pole and push into it. However I'll work through every position I can think of including bear hugging with both arms, with one arm, with one arm and support from the other arm similar to a headlock, squeezing into the chest or shoulders, standing all the way up down to all the way kneeling and even lying down, or seated bear hug and of course squeezing or twisting and pulling or pushing forward and back.

Log Chain Isometrics

Using a chain or rope or cable is a great way to do isometrics and was practiced by some of the greats like Alexander Zaas and Bruce Lee. It's an easy way to carry around something you can do a lot of the isometrics I've already shown in the course if you're traveling. In fact my friend, Bud Jeffries, carries one around when he's touring performing strongman shows, but this is a little different idea.

What I've done here is take a heavy logging chain and attach it to any immoveable object. The idea is to pull the chain, which is long and fairly heavy, tight. This provides a surprising amount of resistance and it's a lot harder than it looks. I then hold it with that tension on it and do multiple direction movements while I'm holding the isometric contraction with the chain. I do this either for the direct muscle that I'm holding with like in holding a bicep curl. I keep the bicep contracted and locked there and then move my arm and body in many different directions, up and down, side to side and in circles so that I'm working that one muscle and all the surrounding muscles super hard. Or I'll do a pull or push that activates my whole body like pulling to the side and squatting down and twisting and then make those same up and down, side to side and circular motions. You can do small motions or large ones. You can go deliberately slow or intentionally fast, one hand or two. One of the great things is you can switch back and forth from exercises without stopping – you just have to change your body angle so when one muscle gets tired you switch to another angle and keep going.

Editor's Note: This has similarities to Battling Ropes which was invented by another great strongman, Jon Brookfield. It's different however in that Battling Ropes is done with slack purposely in the rope or chain and whipping motions to create a wave that runs the length of the rope. This is done with high tension held the entire time and then motions to accentuate the muscle and tension in the body. Hope this helps everyone understand.

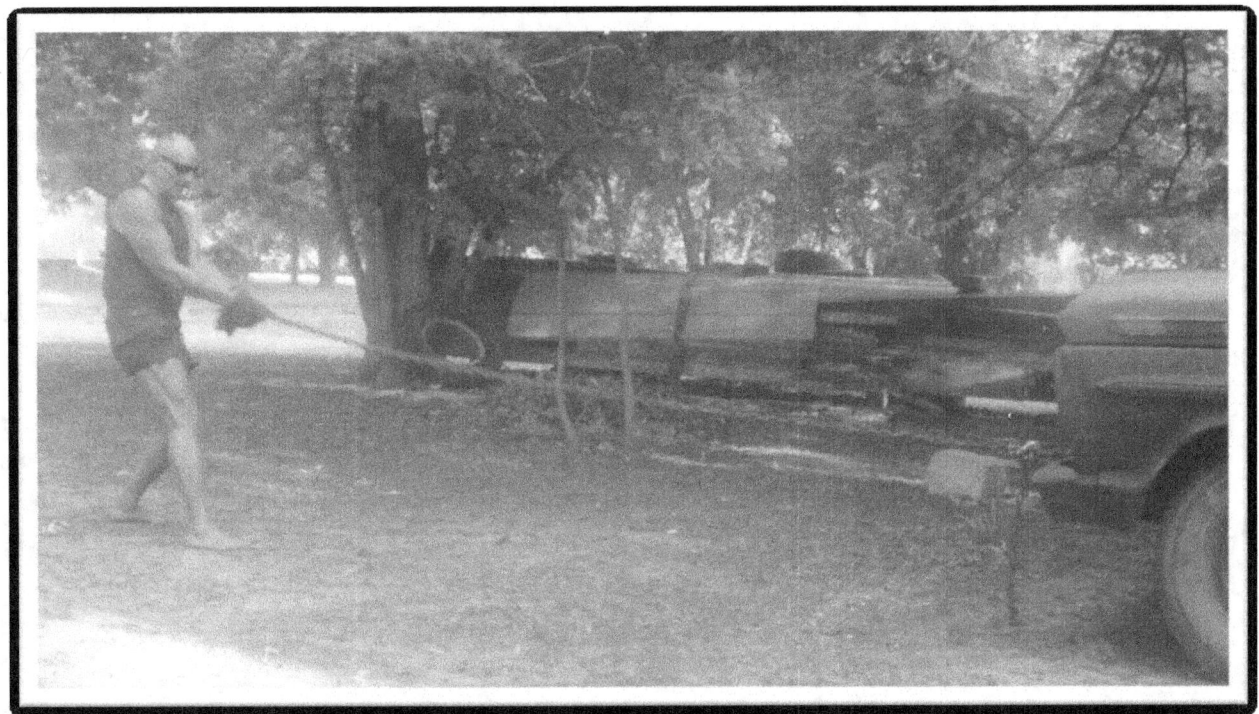

Straight pull back, standing with side to side swing

Straight Pull back, kneeling with circle motion

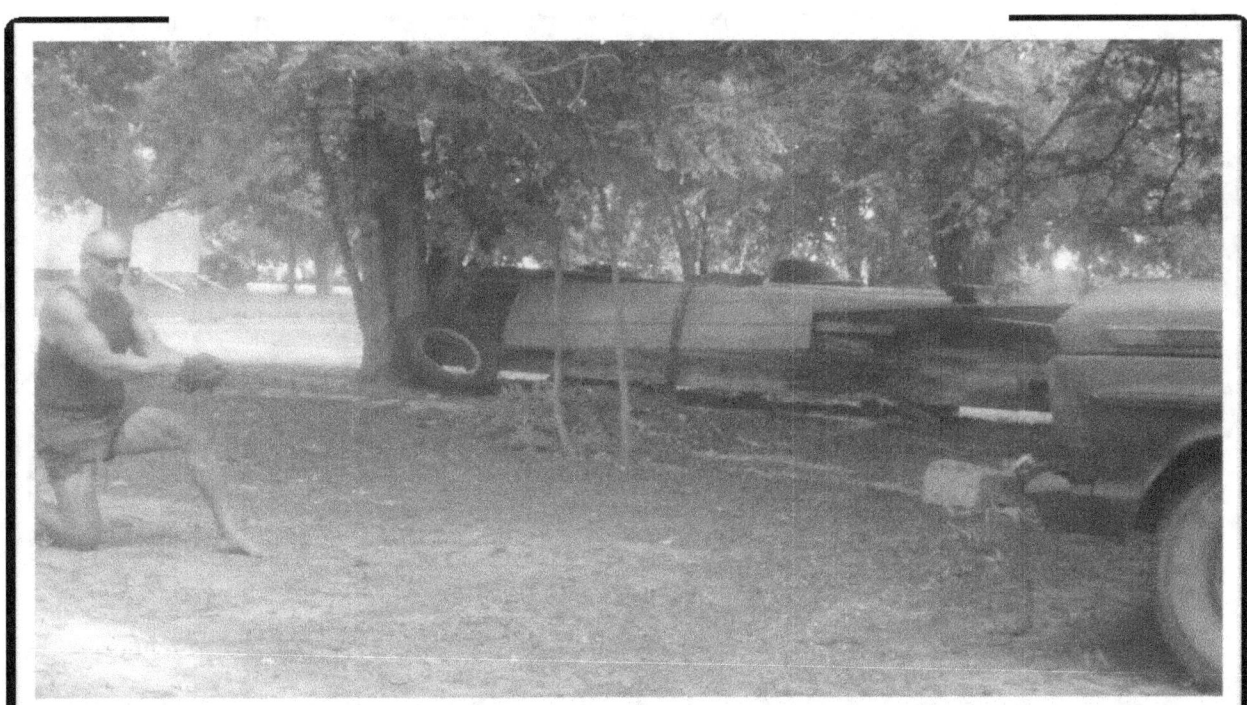

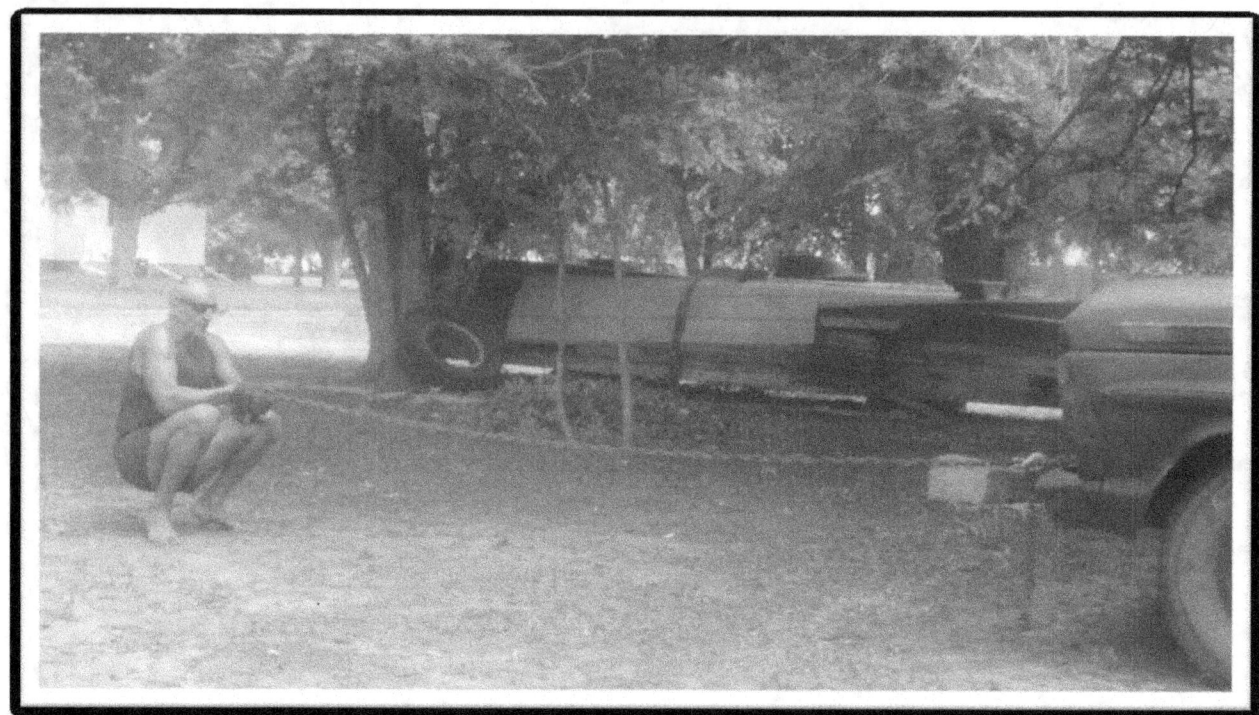

Straight pull back in squat with up and down motion

Twisting Pull back in full squat in Jerk Reps motion

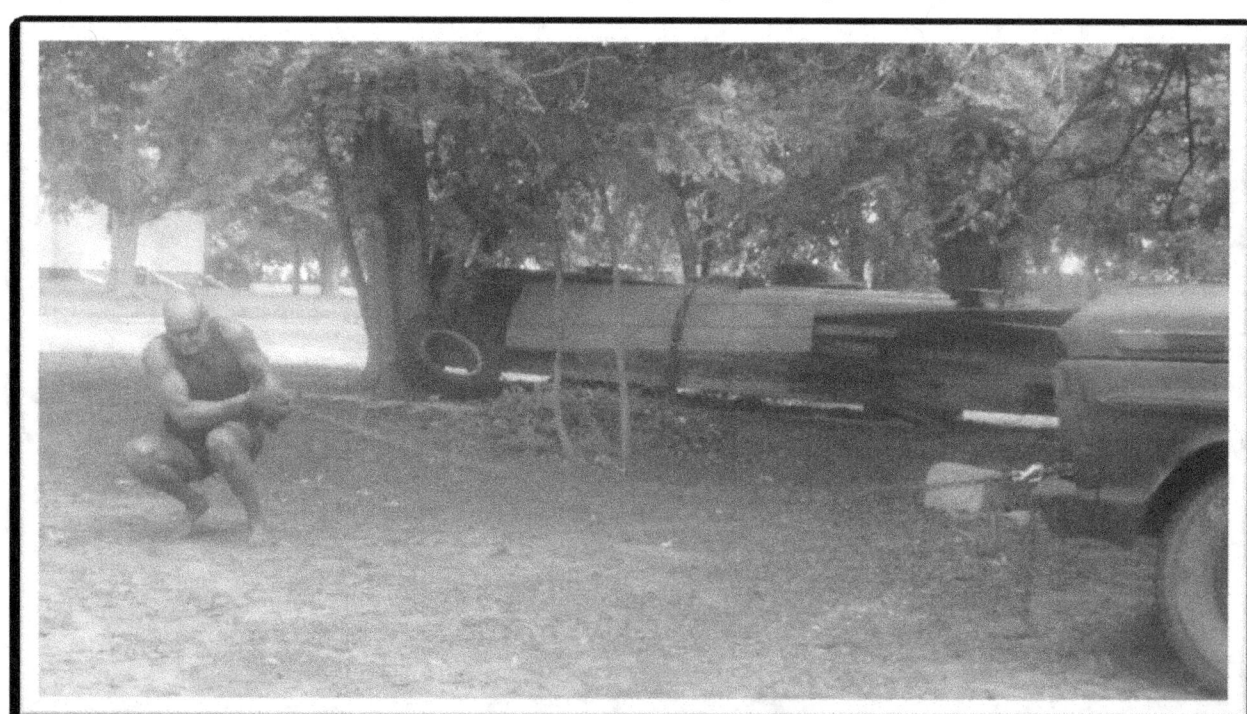

Body Against Body Self Resistance and the Pliers Workout

To me one of the great things about isometrics is that you can literally do them at an time. Included in isometrics to me, in my definition are two styles the old timers used that some people might not think of as a regular isometric. One is muscle control which is literally flexing individual muscles. The other is self-resistance which is what Charles Atlas used to do in his isometrics course. What I do is really a combination of both. I like to do individual muscle flexes, by literally tensing a muscle and then letting it go. Sometimes I do this by use of resistance around me, for instance one hand pushing against the other or your feet on the ground twisting and pushing into the ground or your hands or feet pushing against a chair you're sitting in.

By pushing or pulling against something you give yourself something to focus on while you're flexing that particular muscle. One of the ways I've done this is to use a pair of pliers to squeeze. While I'm squeezing them do different motions of flexing my upper body muscles. This is a combination of dynamic tension and muscle control using the pliers to help everything fire by squeezing them. It works your grip like crazy and you can concentrate on any muscle by simply pulling your arm into the position that flexes that muscle. For instance you want to work the bicep, squeeze the pliers and flex your arm like you're doing a curl. From there I keep the muscle contracted and then move my arm around in circles in forward or back or into lots of different positions that keep my bicep flexed in many different angles. You can do this for the tricep, chest, shoulders and back as well. I also like to flex my wrist and move it around in different patterns and circles while I'm doing this and going from position to position such as my arm held out in front or off to the side or over head. You can get a tremendous burn in the muscle and really work it that way. Plus you really get your mind in touch with the muscles by doing this which makes them stronger.

I like to do this in different positions flexing my leg muscles and twisting, my abdominal muscles and twisting, pushing and giving self resistance in many angles to my neck so I work everything from head to toe.

Flexing my leg and twisting in and out to do self resistance.

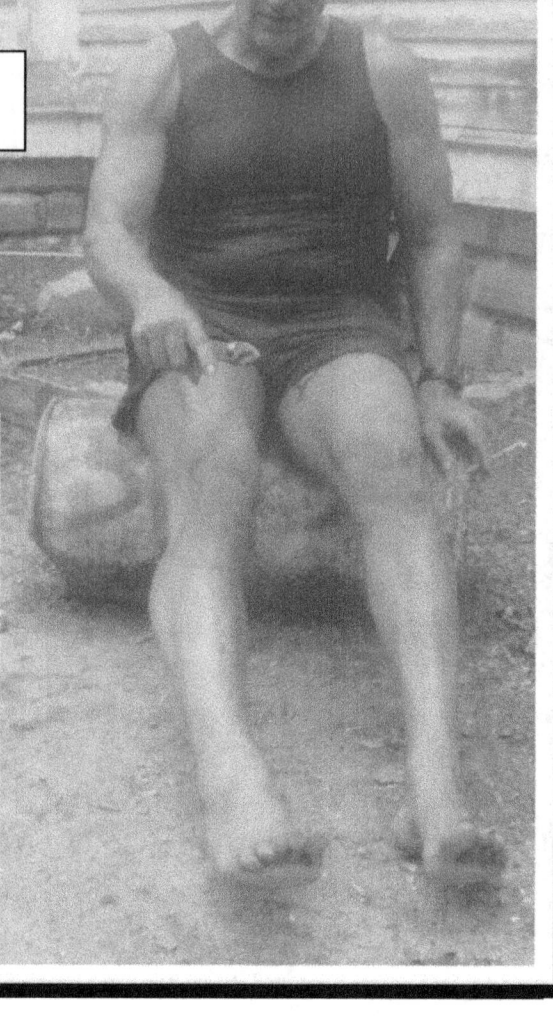

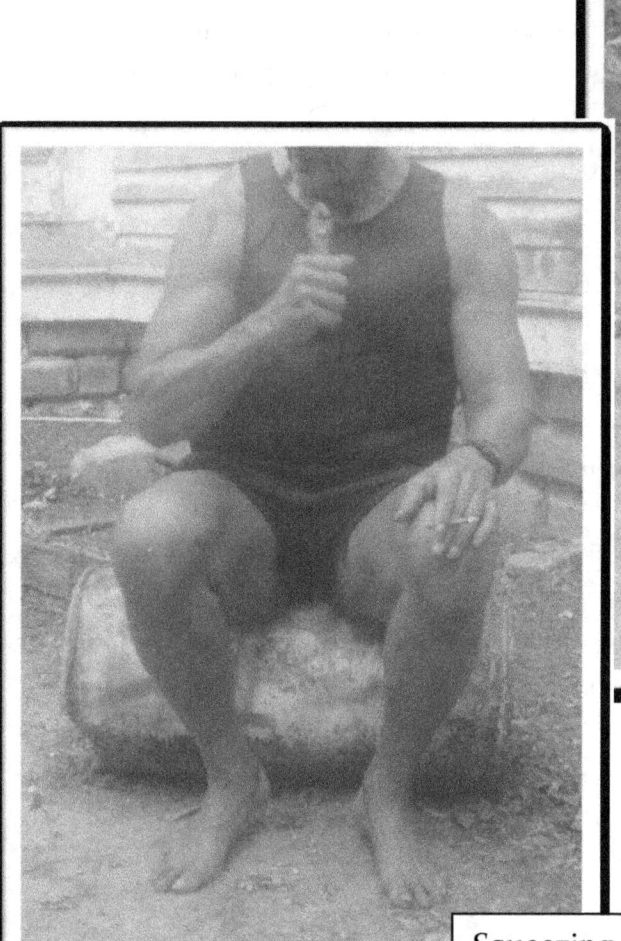

Squeezing pliers to do my combination of self resistance and muscle control isometrics. Here I'm holding the top of a hammer curl position squeezing the bicep and flexing my wrist back and forth.

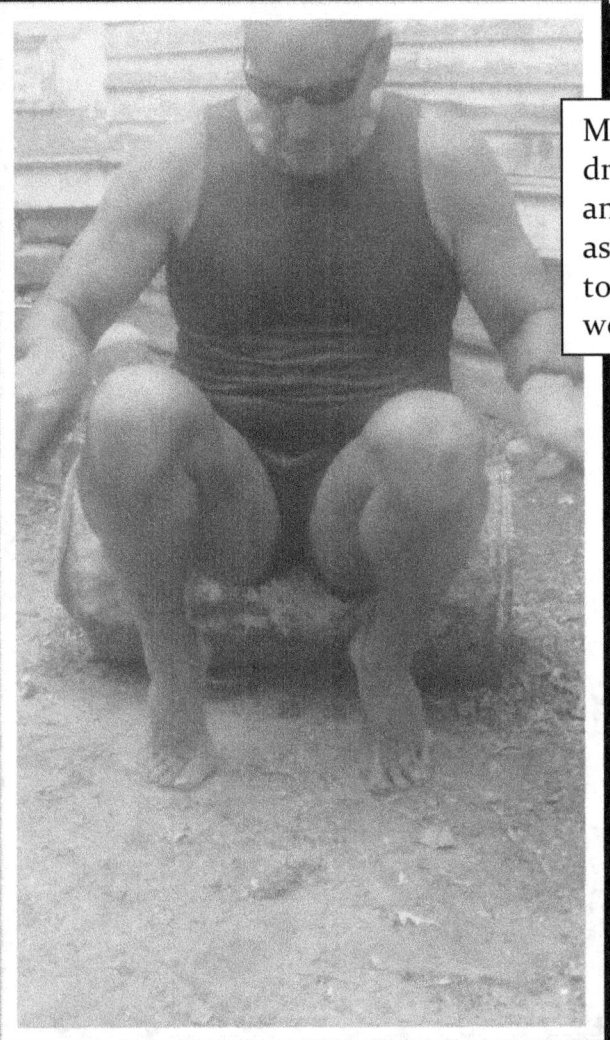

More self resistance here by driving my toes into the ground and twisting in and out as well as forcing my knees in and out to work the thigh muscles as well.

Here I'm squeezing the pliers while twisting my wrist and making circular motions concentrating on flexing the bicep and shoulder muscles.

Heavy Equipment Isometrics and Testing Your Strength

You all know I live in Nebraska which is farm country. One of the types of strength that's very important to me is the kind a farmer or laborer would use. My real training these days is isometrics almost exclusively, but I want to test that strength regularly and see what I'm getting out of my training. Also, farm equipment and heavy machinery make great isometric tools. They almost always give you odd angles to push and pull from and give you a goal. If you can't move it today maybe if you keep doing isometrics with it, may one day you will pick it up. So I regularly find things I can't lift and keep trying till I can.

Here are a few pictures of that:

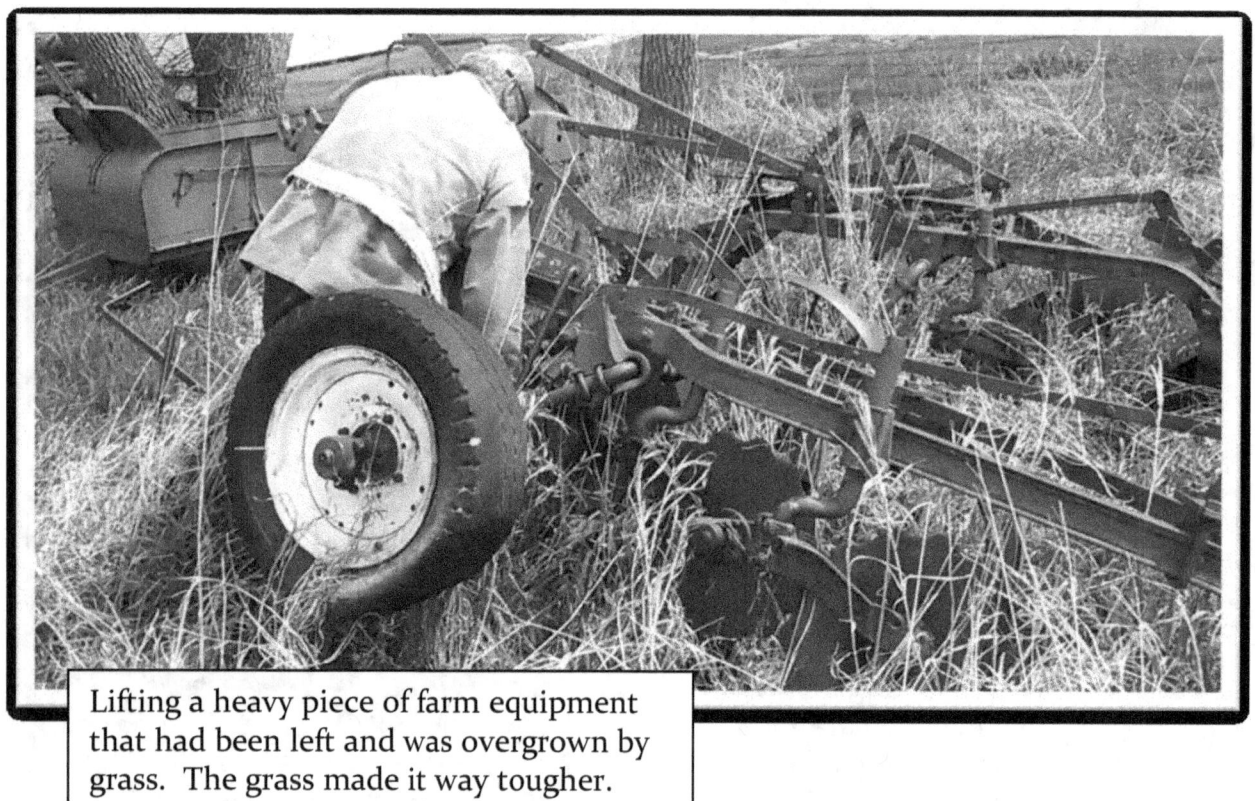

Lifting a heavy piece of farm equipment that had been left and was overgrown by grass. The grass made it way tougher.

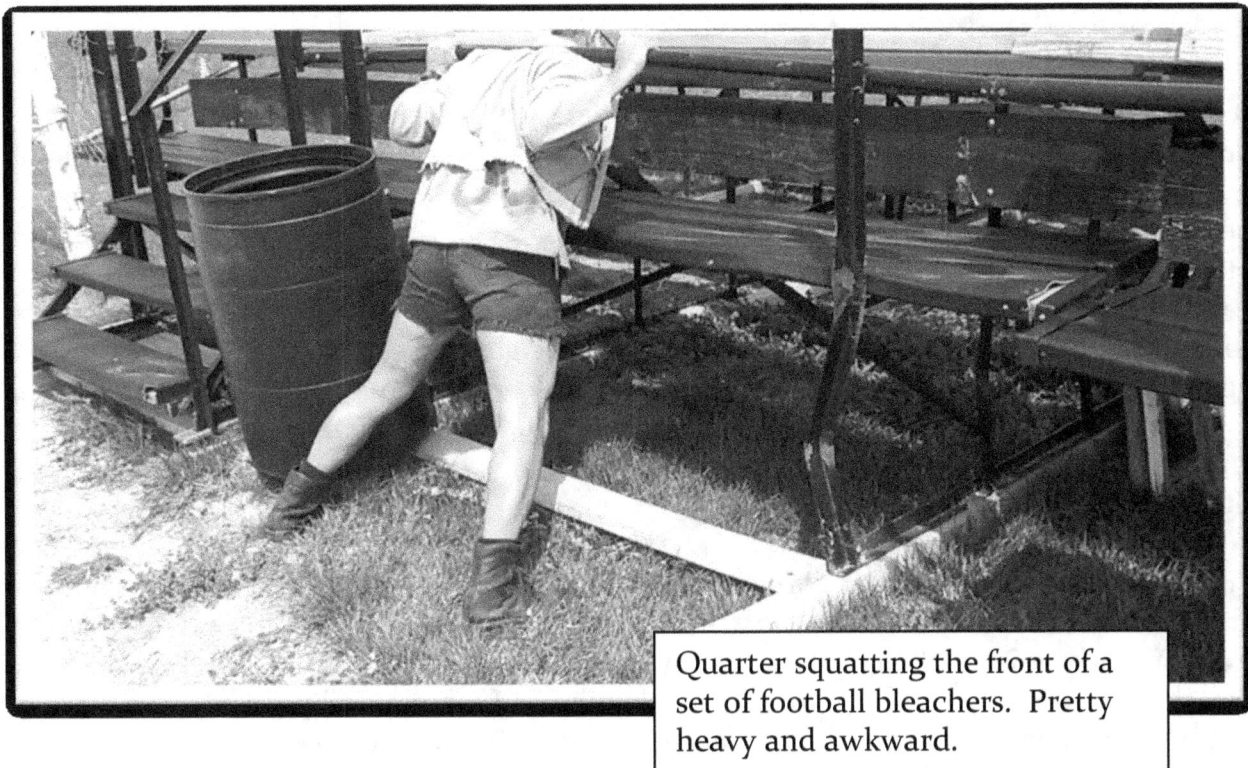

Quarter squatting the front of a set of football bleachers. Pretty heavy and awkward.

Lifting the side and back of a fertilizer tank and trailer.

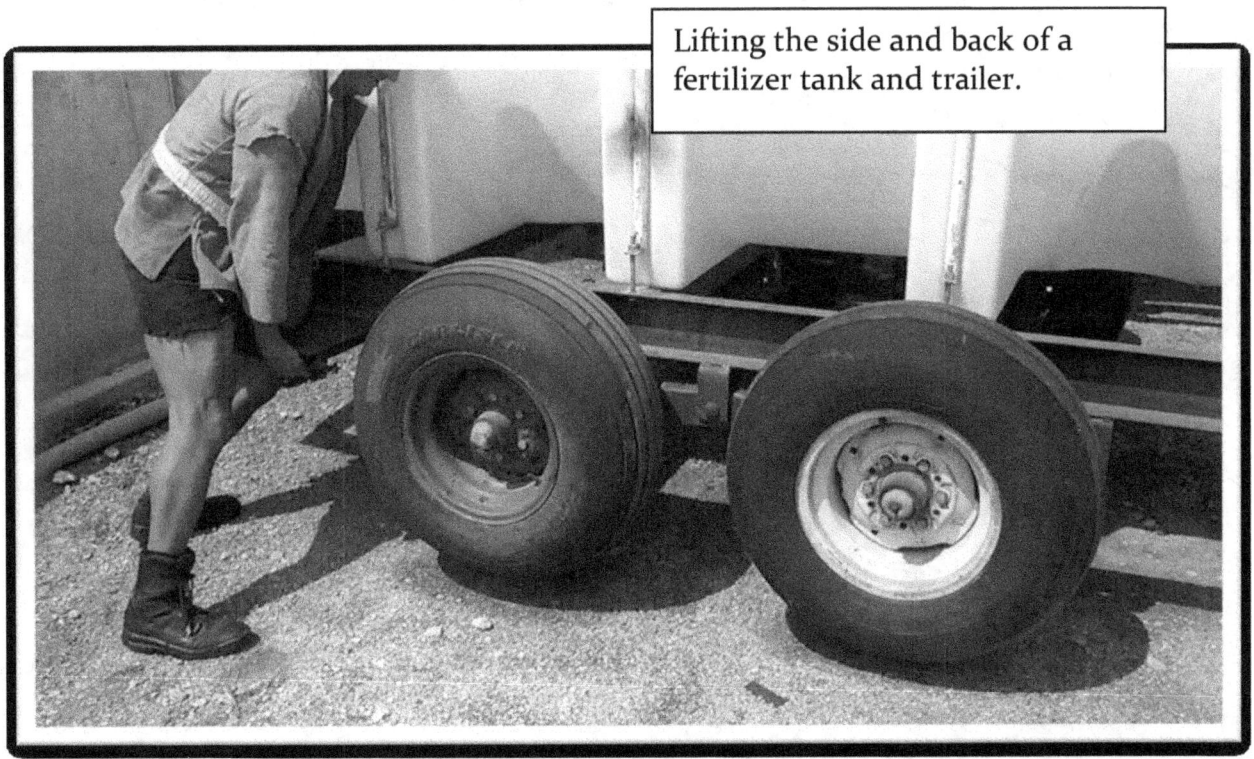

If I Had It To Do Over

If I was to start all over again and become strong, I'd definitely avoid eating like a horse and pushing my bodyweight super high and doing low reps with extremely heavy weights without being in great condition as well. Even if you become stronger this way, it's absolutely not worth it to ruin your health. Instead, I'd do isometrics mixed with the Heavy Iron. Also, instead of increasing the weight quickly, I'd increase the number of sets each time I do a specific exercise. So, if I start with 3 sets of 2 reps, I'd like to gradually get to perhaps, 40 sets of 2 reps before I increase the weight and start with 3 sets of 2 reps again. This kind of training will increase your bodily energy, toughen tendons, ligaments, joints and nerves. Even though you need to be careful with isometrics when you are just starting out, the chances to hurt yourself are very slim compared to sports or weight lifting.

I'd recommend if you want **to gain bodyweight** through isometrics, you'd need to do shorter workouts will more intensity, shorter holds and reps.
To lose bodyweight through isometrics, you'll want to train a couple of hours per day. In just three weeks, you'll change your body completely. In fact, you'll probably lose weight faster than using anything else, while keeping your strength and speed.

Because of its safety and the incredible results I've gotten, I'd concentrate very heavily on the isometrics and stay much leaner but be just as strong. For all you out there doing heavy training and isometrics, I respect you and wish you the best and I hope to hear from you and that this training helps you. So keep getting super strong and healthy and tell them the High Plains, Heavy Metal Iron Master showed you a few cool things.

Train Hard!

Steve Justa

Notes

www.ingramcontent.com/pod-product-compliance
Lightning Source LLC
Chambersburg PA
CBHW080432290526

45791CB00008BA/2472